Techniques of measurement in medicine: 3
Series Editor: Dr B. Watson
Department of Medical Electronics
St Bartholomew's Hospital, London
Consultant Editor: Professor J. Rotblat

Radionuclide techniques in medicine

Radionuclide techniques in medicine

JOAN M. McALISTER

Cambridge University Press
CAMBRIDGE
LONDON - NEW YORK - MELBOURNE

Published by the Syndics of the Cambridge University Press
The Pitt Building, Trumpington Street, Cambridge CB2 1RP
Bentley House, 200 Euston Road, London NW1 2DB
32 East 57th Street, New York, NY 10022, USA
296 Beaconsfield Parade, Middle Park, Melbourne 3206, Australia

First published 1979

Printed in Great Britain at the University Press, Cambridge

Library of Congress Cataloguing in Publication Data

McAlister, Joan M.
Radionuclide techniques in medicine.

(Techniques of measurement in medicine; 3)
Includes bibliographical references and index.
1. Nuclear medicine. I. Title. II. Series.
[DNLM: 1. Radioisotopes – Diagnostic use.
2. Technology, Radiologic. WN445 M114r]
R895.M33 616.07'575 78-68348

ISBN 0 521 22402 0 hard covers
ISBN 0 521 29474 6 paperback

To my sister Betty, without whom this book would not have been written

Contents

Foreword

During the last thirty years the use of radioactive isotopes in medicine has increased at a rapid pace. The ready availability of a large range of radioactive pharmaceuticals led to an increase in applications, but the development of detectors and the associated electronic equipment has played the major role.

The early Geiger counters were quickly replaced by scintillation counters, the latter having the advantage of easy discrimination between isotopes as well as improving the limits of detection. The gamma camera was the next major development and enabled the spatial distribution of radioactive substances in the body to be measured. Computer techniques have enhanced the image quality and also enabled dynamic physiological studies to be undertaken.

In a series on techniques of measurement in medicine it was essential that one of the first volumes in the series should be about radioactive isotope measurement techniques, but I realised that for the author it would be a formidable task. I asked Joan McAlister to undertake this task because for twenty years she was head of the Isotope Department at St Bartholomew's Hospital, and I had seen her apply this new technology with meticulous care. Professor Rotblat was one of the early pioneers in the use of isotopes in medicine and therefore there has been even closer interaction between the Consultant Editor and the author on this occasion. We all hope that this book will be a source of information for all those scientists, technicians and doctors who are routinely using radioactive isotopes for both in-vivo and in-vitro studies in medicine and the life sciences.

Bernard W. Watson

Acknowledgements

My thanks are due to Dr Bernard Watson for asking me to write this book and for helpful guidance, and to Professor J. Rotblat for advice and constructive criticism.

I am grateful to all my colleagues, past and present, technicians, physicists and clinicians, who have contributed to the work of the Radioisotope Department of St Bartholomew's Hospital, and thereby to the writing of this book. It is impossible to name them all, but special thanks are due to Laurie Hawkins, Cyril Nimmon, Sophie Ostrowski, Peter Jarritt, Jagdish Mistry, Clifton West and Clarkson Prescott for their interest, helpful criticism, and assistance in providing material for many of the diagrams, and to Keith Britton and Alex Elliott for useful comments after reading the typescript. Many other colleagues have given willing help in different ways, including John Callow, Tony Goddard, John Mallard, Sidney Osborn and Peter Turner.

Most of the diagrams and photographs have been prepared by the Department of Medical Illustration, St Bartholomew's Hospital, for which I must thank David Tredinnick and Julie Dorrington. I would also like to express my appreciation of the financial support provided by Baird-Atomic Ltd for the reproduction of the colour photographs in Fig. 9.7.

Finally, I am greatly indebted to my secretary, Miss Lilian Murkin, for much patient work in typing the earlier drafts, and some of the later ones, and to Miss Grover for much of the later typing.

1. Introduction

The application of radionuclides to medical diagnosis and treatment has a relatively short history. The phenomenon of radioactivity was originally discovered by Henri Becquerel in 1896, and Pierre and Marie Curie isolated the naturally occurring element radium in 1899. The use of radium in the treatment of malignant disease was first introduced at the turn of the century, and was well established by 1920. It was not until 1938, however, that the discovery of nuclear fission made possible the subsequent development of the nuclear reactor, and the large-scale production of artificial radioactive nuclides. It was immediately realised that the latter opened up great possibilities in the medical field. The radioactive isotope was chemically indistinguishable from the stable isotopes of the element, but minute quantities of it in the body could be detected externally by virtue of the radiation it emitted; it could therefore be used as a 'tracer' to follow the metabolism of a substance through the body. The obvious example was the radioactive isotope of iodine. Iodine is metabolised exclusively by the thyroid gland, and if radioactive iodine was administered either by mouth or by injection the amount taken up by the thyroid gland could be measured, as could the amount subsequently released into the blood as thyroid hormone. Moreover, since the radioactivity concentrates in the thyroid gland it could be used to treat the overactive gland in hyperthyroidism, or the malignant gland in thyroid carcinoma.

When the author came to St Bartholomew's Hospital in 1957 the work in the Radioisotope Department was confined to the use of radioactive iodine in the form of iodine-131, for the diagnosis of thyroid dysfunction and its treatment. The only equipment available was a ring of Geiger counters and two hand-operated portable scintillation counters. There has been a spectacular growth over the past 20 years from these very simple techniques to extremely sophisticated ones. At the present time, about 20 different radiopharmaceuticals are being used in the Department of Nuclear Medicine and Radioisotopes, and studies involving most organs of the body are being carried out, in collaboration with nearly every medical and surgical department in the hospital. The applications have been much wider than was originally conceived. Apart from the true 'tracer' techniques, which necessitate a radioactive isotope or isotopically-labelled compound which is chemically identical with the element under investigation, many other techniques have been developed. The imaging techniques are those in most widespread use. They involve using a radiopharmaceutical which is taken up specifically by the organ, or tissue, under investigation, but is not necessarily a physiological substance. The distribution of the material is determined by measurement of the radioactivity. Dynamic studies are also carried out, for example to investigate kidney function, blood flow and cardiac function; with these studies the radiopharmaceuticals must also behave in a physiological manner, but are not necessarily true tracers.

The rapid progress in imaging techniques is illustrated in Figs. 1.1 to 1.5. The earliest imaging was of the thyroid gland. Fig. 1.1 shows the type of result obtained in 1948 by Ansell & Rotblat using Geiger-counter equipment for point-by-point counting. Scintillation counters were first used for brain imaging in 1952. Figs. 1.2 to 1.5 show the development over the years 1955 to 1977. Allen & Risser, in 1955, used an automatic scanner to produce the result shown in Fig. 1.2 after injection of ^{131}I-labelled human serum albumin; they interpreted this as a positive result demonstrating cerebral metastases which were confirmed at autopsy. The IDL (Isotope Developments Ltd) automatic scanner first used at St Bartholomew's Hospital in 1964 is shown in Fig. 1.3, with a positive result obtained after injection of ^{99m}Tc pertechnetate. The more sophisticated purpose-built brain scanner developed by J & P Engineering (Reading) Ltd in 1971 is shown in Fig. 1.4, with the positive brain scan result. A further development of that equipment is the J & P tomographic scanner referred to in Chapter 7. Fig. 1.5 shows brain images obtained with a modern gamma camera, which is described in Chapter 7 (Fig. 7.16*a*).

The developments described have been achieved through an understanding of the nature of radioactivity and the radiations emitted, and of the requirements for obtaining accurate measurements and adequate sensitivity and resolution, as well as by technological advances. It is very important that the fundamental principles, which apply equally to simple tests and sophisticated investigations, are fully understood by workers in the field. It is of no use, for example, to employ advanced computer technology to process results, if the experimental data which are fed into the computer are not based on sound scientific principles, or to use expensive imaging equipment if it is not operated under optimum conditions, or if the radiopharmaceutical used does not conform to the necessary standard or serve the required physiological function. This book aims at explaining these fundamental principles, and how they are applied in practical techniques.

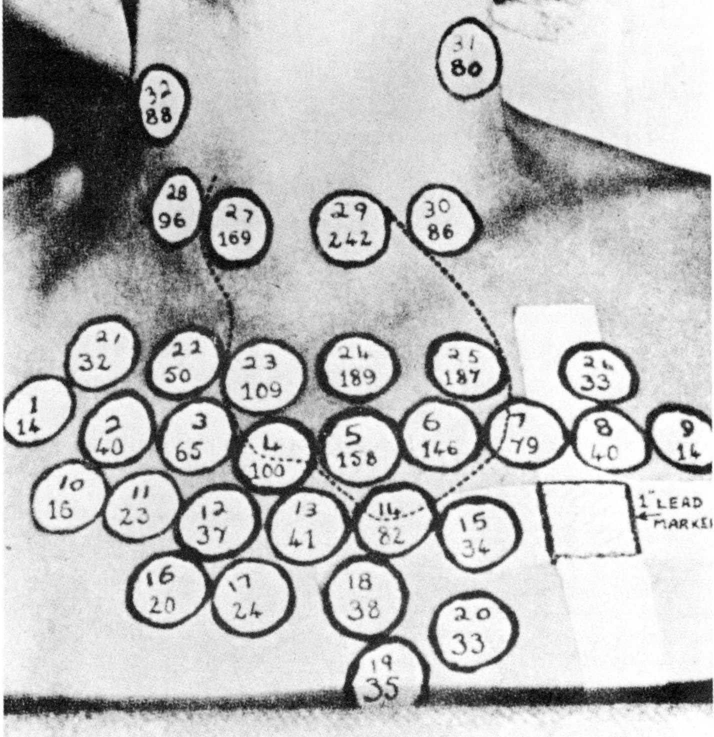

Fig. 1.1. Thyroid image obtained with Geiger counter equipment used by Ansell & Rotblat in 1948. (Reproduced from *Br. J. Radiol.* (1948), **21**, 552–8, by kind permission of the authors and editors.)

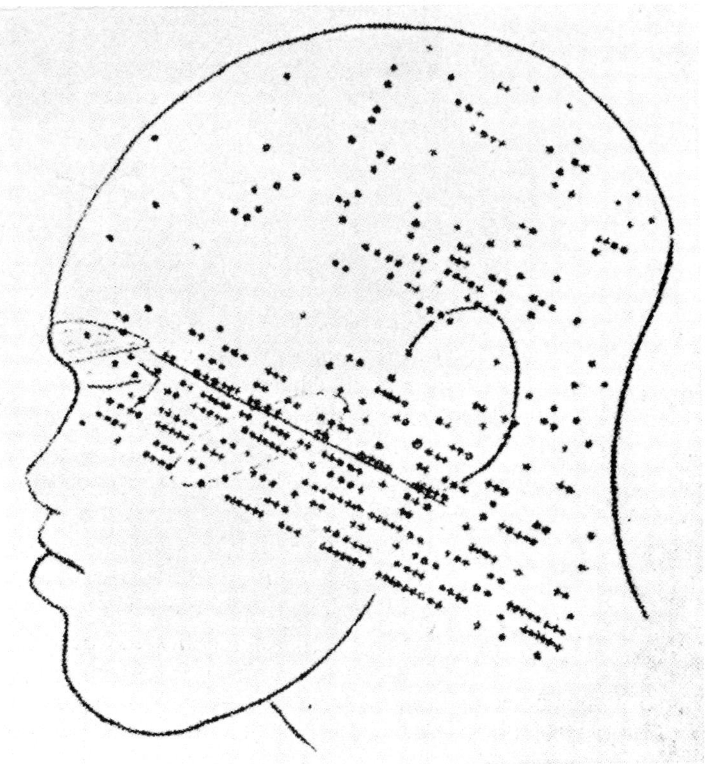

Fig. 1.2. Brain scan obtained by Allen & Risser in 1955. (Reproduced from *Br. J. Radiol.* (1973), **46**, 889–98, by kind permission of the authors and editors.)

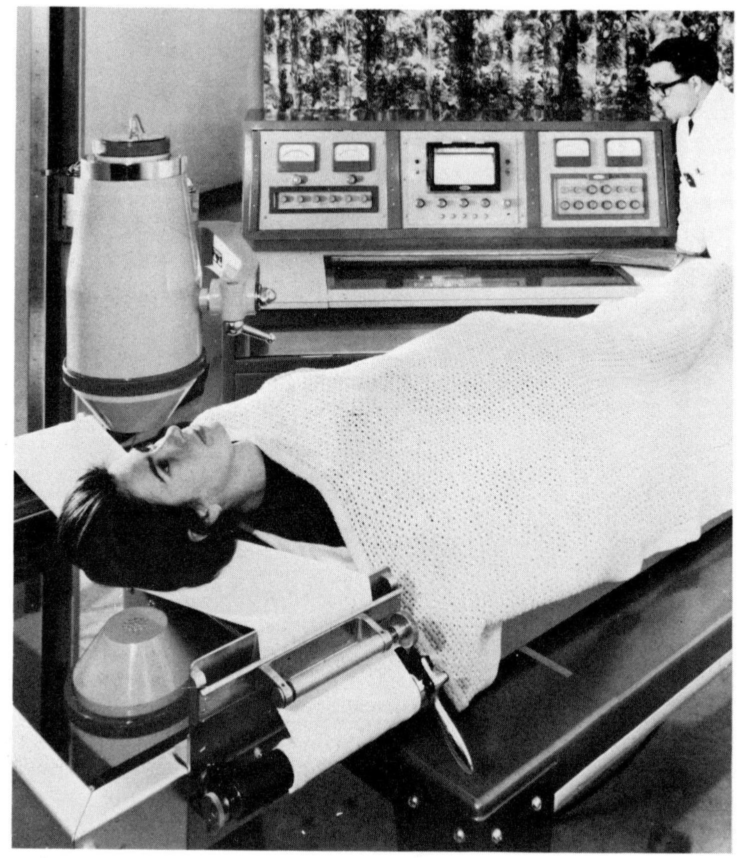

(a)

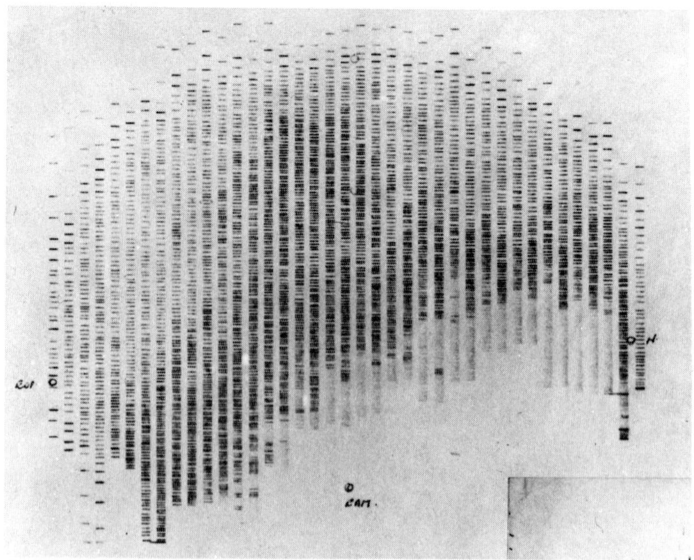

(b)

Fig. 1.3. (*a*) IDL automatic scanner installed at St Bartholomew's Hospital in 1964. (*b*) Brain scan obtained with equipment shown in (*a*).

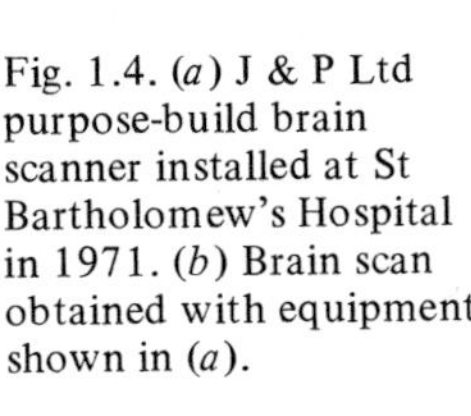

Fig. 1.4. (*a*) J & P Ltd purpose-build brain scanner installed at St Bartholomew's Hospital in 1971. (*b*) Brain scan obtained with equipment shown in (*a*).

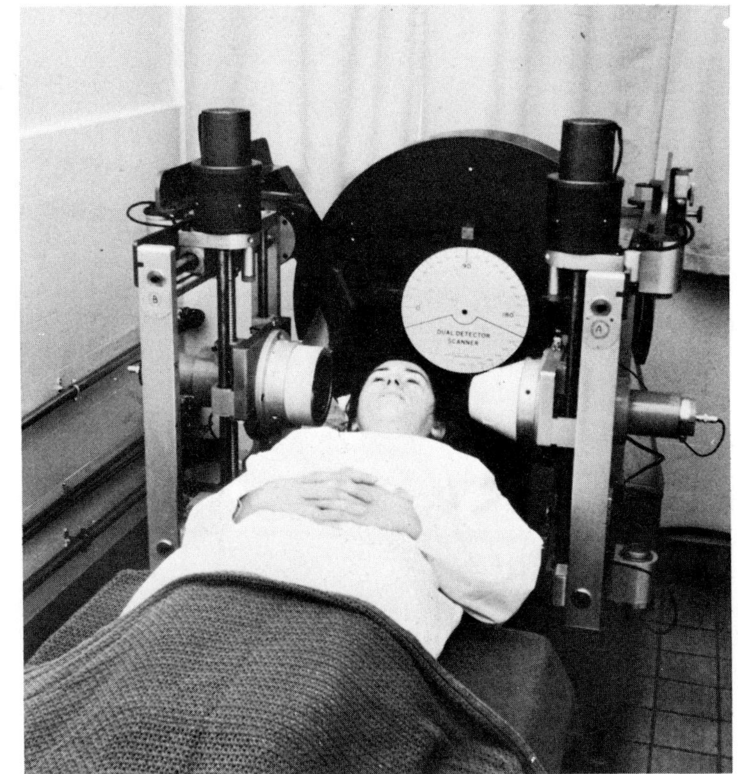

(*a*)

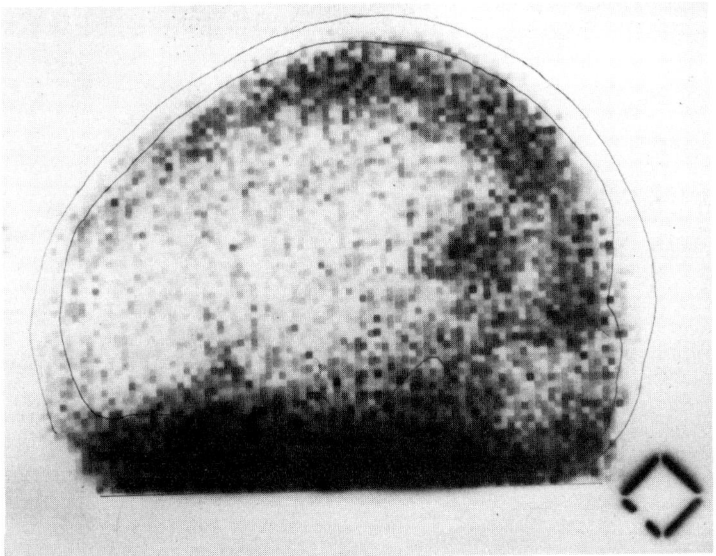

(*b*)

Fig. 1.5. Brain scintigrams obtained with modern gamma camera.

Right lateral

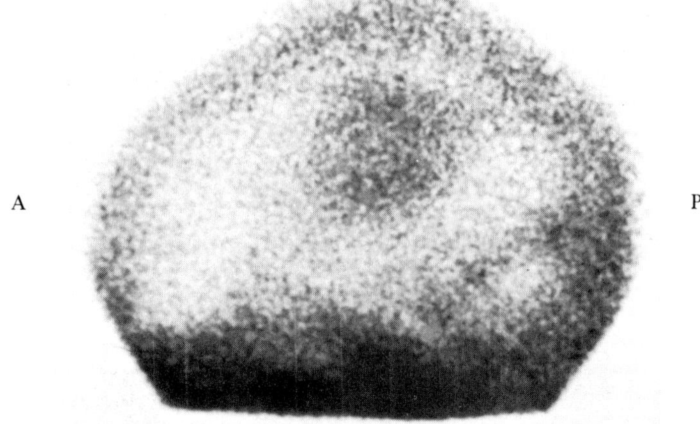

Posterior

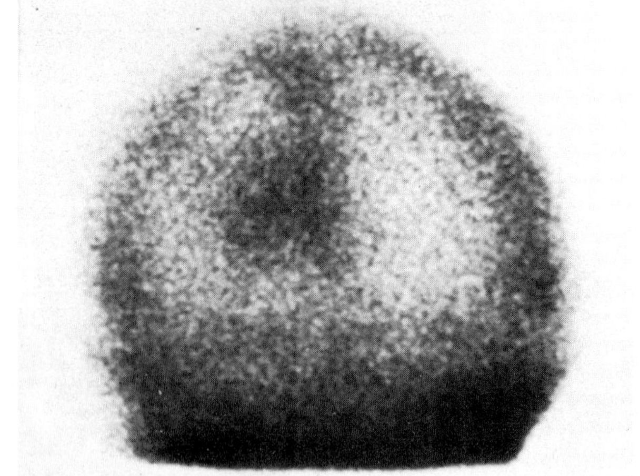

2. Radioactivity, ionising radiations and radiation exposure

Radioactivity

In order to understand fully the nature of radioactivity it is necessary to know something of the structure of the atom; this is dealt with in Chapter 10, and the terms are defined in the Glossary. A brief account is given here in order that the reader may comprehend the chapters that follow.

All matter is composed of elements, such as hydrogen, carbon, oxygen, copper, etc., each of which has well-defined chemical properties. Atoms are the units of the elements, and each atom has a nucleus which contains positively charged protons and uncharged neutrons, and is surrounded by a number of negatively charged orbital electrons. The number of protons in the nucleus, referred to as the atomic number (Z), determines the nature of the element. The number of orbital electrons is equal to the number of protons, and the electrons are involved in chemical reactions. Thus for any one element the atomic number is always the same; for hydrogen it is 1, for carbon 6, for oxygen 8 and for iodine 53.

The number of protons plus neutrons determines the mass of the atom and is referred to as the mass number (A); the number of neutrons is not necessarily the same for all atoms in an element. A nuclide is a species of atom having a unique atomic number and a unique mass number. Any element may contain more than one nuclide, that is it may have more than one species of atom, and these are referred to as isotopes of that element. All isotopes of an element have the same atomic number, which is characteristic of the element, but each has its unique mass number which is different from that of other isotopes. Since the chemical properties of an element are determined by its atomic number, isotopes are chemically indistinguishable. The element oxygen as it occurs in nature has three isotopes, all with atomic number 8, and with, respectively, mass numbers of 16, 17 and 18; each of the three isotopes is a nuclide. The composition of a nuclide can be denoted by the atomic number as a subscript to the chemical symbol and the mass number as a superscript: e.g. ${}^{16}_{8}O$, ${}^{17}_{8}O$ and ${}^{18}_{8}O$. However, since the symbol of the element is itself characteristic of the atomic number, the subscript is usually omitted: e.g. ${}^{16}O$, ${}^{17}O$ and ${}^{18}O$. Since chemical properties are dependent on the atomic number, the three isotopes of oxygen are chemically indistinguishable.

It is possible to produce by artificial means isotopes of an element that have greater or fewer numbers of neutrons in their nuclei than do the stable isotopes, and which are therefore unstable. These are radioactive isotopes; the atoms are continuously disintegrating, with the emission of ionising radiation. As a result of the process of disintegration the substance changes into a different element: e.g. ^{15}O is a radioactive nuclide which is an isotope of oxygen; it disintegrates to form nitrogen, ^{15}N.

Modes of disintegration

There are three main primary disintegration processes that are encountered in medical work; they are beta-emission (β-emission), positron-emission (β^+-emission) and electron capture (K-capture).

In β-emission the radioactive nuclide, the nucleus of which has too many neutrons, changes to the (usually) stable nuclide one place higher in the Periodic Table, with the emission of an electron (β-particle) of maximum energy specific for that disintegration.

β^+-emission takes place in radioactive nuclides in which the nuclei have too few neutrons; the nuclide changes to the (usually) stable nuclide one place lower in the Periodic Table, with the emission of a positron (positively charged electron) of energy specific to that disintegration. The positron, however, is an unstable particle and is almost immediately annihilated in combination with an electron to form two quanta of annihilation radiation. These are gamma radiations of energy 0.51 MeV each; they are emitted in exactly opposite directions from the point at which the positron is annihilated. Coincidence circuitry may be used to detect the two opposing quanta.

In electron capture the nucleus captures one orbital electron from the atom and, as in β^+ decay, the nuclide changes to a nuclide which belongs to an element one place down in the Periodic Table. The atom is left in an excited state, and it reverts to its ground state with emission of characteristic X-radiation. The disintegration process of electron capture is detected by means of the characteristic X-radiation.

Each of these three main processes may leave the nucleus in an excited state, which causes it to emit γ-radiation. In some instances the nucleus does not emit the γ-radiation immediately, but with an observable half-life which may be as long as a few hours. It is then said to be in a metastable state, denoted by the letter m after the mass number, and to decay by isomeric transition. An important example is technetium-99m (^{99m}Tc).

The manner in which a radionuclide disintegrates is shown

diagrammatically as a disintegration scheme which details the type and energy of the radiations emitted; these are invariable for any particular nuclide. Examples are shown in Chapter 10.

Disintegration rate and half-life
The rate at which a radionuclide disintegrates is characterised by its decay constant. Radioactive decay is an exponential process, that is the rate of decay is proportional to the amount of the substance present. It can be shown mathematically that the time taken for the amount of a radioactive substance to be decreased to one-half of its original value is always constant; this time is referred to as its half-life ($T_{\frac{1}{2}}$). It follows that after one $T_{\frac{1}{2}}$ the amount is reduced to 50% of its original value, after two $T_{\frac{1}{2}}$ it is reduced to 25% (50% of 50%), after three $T_{\frac{1}{2}}$ to 12½%, and so on, in theory never quite reaching zero but being reduced to less than 1% after seven $T_{\frac{1}{2}}$.

Units
The old unit of activity is the curie (Ci); it is defined as the amount of a radioactive substance which gives rise to 3.7×10^{10} disintegrations per second. The millicurie (mCi) and the microcurie (μCi) are, respectively, one-thousandth and one-millionth of a curie. The new SI unit of activity is the becquerel (Bq); it corresponds to 1 disintegration per second. Thus, 1 μCi equals 3.7×10^4 Bq; conversion tables are given in Chapter 10. In this book both the old unit and its SI equivalent are used.

Ionising radiations

The term ionising radiations is a general one, used to describe radiations which produce ions, that is pairs of negatively and positively charged particles, in the material through which they pass. The radiations are detected by means of the ions produced. It is important that the worker knows the properties of the different radiations, has some concept of radiation exposure, absorbed dose and dose equivalent, and is familiar with the units in which they are expressed. This is necessary in order to understand the methods of measurement, the problems of radiation hazards involved, and the reasons for radiation protection measures. A brief general account is given here, and the reader is referred to Chapter 11 for the physics.

The types of radiation most commonly encountered when handling radionuclides in the medical field are β-, X-, and γ-radiation.

β-radiation

β-radiation is a stream of electrons, which produces ions directly. It is absorbed very easily, with the result that all its energy is deposited within a small volume, giving rise to a localised high radiation dose. The energies of the β-particles vary from zero to a maximum which is given in the disintegration scheme; the average energy is about one-third of the maximum. The range of β-radiation is dependent on its energy, and also on the material through which it is passing. It should be appreciated that β-radiation with maximum energy up to 0.3 MeV will be completely absorbed in 1 mm of polystyrene. It follows that if a radioactive solution emitting this kind of radiation is contained in a vial or syringe, the radiation will not penetrate the walls of the container, and therefore will pose no problem. However, if the same solution is spilt on the skin, the β-radiation can give rise to a localised high radiation dose. It is for this reason that gloves must be worn when handling any unsealed radioactive source of strength greater than 0.1 μCi ml^{-1} (3.7 kBq ml^{-1}), and even of lower concentration if the volume is large. The quantitative aspects of β-radiation dosimetry are given in Chapter 11.

γ-radiation and X-radiation

γ- and X-radiation are electromagnetic radiations; they do not ionise directly but via the production of secondary electrons. The distinction between γ- and X-radiation relates to their origin; from the point of view of radiation protection they may be considered together, and will be referred to jointly as γ-radiation, except where the text refers specifically to X-radiation.

Attenuation coefficient. γ-radiation is absorbed by matter. The reduction in intensity, or attenuation, of a beam of γ-radiation in any material is dependent on the energy of the radiations, and on the material traversed. Attenuation is exponential (like radioactive decay) and the attenuating power of a material is often expressed in terms of its half-value-thickness or half-value-layer (HVL). One HVL reduces the radiation to 50% of its original intensity, two HVL reduce it to 25%, and so on. Values of HVL for radiations of different energy are given in Chapter 11. It should be noted that lead is an effective screen against radiations, but the effectiveness is reduced at higher energies, and at 2 MeV it takes 1.3 cm of lead to reduce the intensity to one-half.

Inverse square law. γ-radiation, in common with all electromagnetic radiation, obeys the inverse square law; that is, the intensity of radiation is inversely proportional to the square of the distance from a point source. For example, at 20 cm the intensity is one-quarter that at 10 cm. The intensity of γ-radiation (from a radioactive source) to which a worker is exposed may be reduced in two ways: by interposing a lead screen (or screen of other suitable material) between the source and the worker, and by keeping as far away from the source as is practicable.

Speed of handling. In handling any source of radiation the exposure increases with time, and can be reduced by working as quickly as is consistent with taking meticulous care.

Radiation exposure

Any exposure to ionising radiations is assumed to entail a risk of deleterious effects. This risk has been continuously considered by the International Commission on Radiological Protection (ICRP) since its formation in 1928. Its latest publication (ICRP, 1977*b*) recommends a system of dose limitation, which has three main features: that no practice involving radiation exposure shall be adopted unless it gives a positive net benefit; that all exposures shall be kept as low as practicable; and that the 'dose equivalent' to individuals shall not exceed the limits recommended by the Commission. The ICRP give values for the 'dose equivalent limit' (DEL) for the whole body and various tissues, and for the 'annual limits of intake' (ALI) for various nuclides, for radiation workers and for the general public. These values supersede their previous recommendations (ICRP, 1969, 1964, 1965) for maximum permissible body burdens (MPBB) and maximum permissible concentrations in air (MPCa) and in drinking water (MPCw) for different radionuclides. However, the EC Council has adopted the earlier recommendations (EC Council Directive, 1976) and these are therefore mandatory in the EC until the Council formally adopts the 1977 values. Both sets of recommendations are summarised in Table 11.3 (p. 194) and all radiation workers should be familiar with them. All of the references quoted above are given at the end of Chapter 11.

Units of dose equivalent

The 1965 values were expressed in rems, but in Table 11.3 have been converted to sieverts (Sv), the new SI unit of dose equivalent, for comparison with the 1977 values.

Legal requirements

In the UK it is the legal responsibility of employing authorities to ensure that the radiation exposure of all designated workers is regularly monitored and recorded, and that they are kept within the ICRP recommendations. There are also regulations about the storage and disposal of radioactive waste.

Summary

Anyone working with radioactive materials should know:

1. *Concerning radiation protection*

1.1. The legal requirements with regard to radiation exposure and its monitoring.

1.2. The 'local rules' of the institution in which they work.

1.3. The legal requirements with regard to storage and disposal of radioactive materials.

1.4. The emergency procedures in case of accidental spillage.

2. *Concerning the radioactive material being handled*

2.1. Its chemical nature and the symbol of the radioactive nuclide, its atomic number and mass number.

2.2. The disintegration scheme of the nuclide and its half-life.

3. *Concerning the particular sample being handled*

3.1. The activity of the source, in millicuries or microcuries (in SI units, becquerels).

3.2. The volume, and activity per unit volume.

3.3. The reference date, and, with short-lived nuclides, the reference time at which the radioactive content applies.

3.4. The specific activity.

Any radioactive material being dispensed must immediately be given a label showing the radioactive symbol, and the information detailed in 2.1, 3.1, 3.2 and 3.3.

3. Basic instrumentation and sample-counting equipment

Introduction

In radioisotope work the measurements, from a practical point of view, fall into two main categories. The first is the measurement of quantities of radioactive materials. The simplest of these measurements is that of samples of various kinds (for example patient-doses, samples obtained from patients, or samples for in-vitro work); the results can be readily expressed in millicuries or microcuries (gigabecquerels or megabecquerels). Absolute measurement requires complex equipment, and absolute values are obtained by using a calibrated standard instrument. Frequently only relative measurements are required, the absolute value being obtained by comparison with a standardised source. Measurement and localisation of radioactivity within the body are more difficult and require specialised equipment, which will be described in later chapters. The second main category of measurement is that used in radiation protection work, and involves the measurement of radiation exposure-rate or exposure. All of the above measurements are essentially those of radiation emitted, and the fundamental principles of the detectors are the same. However the sensitivity and complexity of the instruments cover a wide range.

The detection and measurement of ionising radiations depend, as is shown in Chapter 11, on the production of ion pairs or of excitation, either directly by particulate radiation such as β-radiation, or indirectly by the production of secondary electrons, in the case of X- or γ-radiation. All radiation detectors are essentially transducers, that is they absorb the radiation and transform it into some form of energy which is readily detectable by conventional means – for example electric current in the case of ionisation chambers and semiconductor devices, electrical pulses in the case of Geiger counters, light photons in the case of scintillation counters, and heat or chemical changes in some specialised detectors. Detectors may be divided into two groups; one, often referred to as pulse detectors, detects individual β-particles or γ-ray interactions, and the other, sometimes referred to as integrating detectors, measures the mean rate of production of ionisation or excitation. Both groups measure *rates* of disintegration or exposure; the term integrating dosemeter is given to an instrument which integrates exposure rate over a period of time to give total exposure.

The various types of detector are considered below.

Ionisation chambers

The earliest type of detector for X- and γ-radiation was the ionisation chamber, which consists essentially of a closed volume of gas and two electrodes across which is maintained an electrical potential difference. The radiation interacts with the material of the wall of the chamber and also with the gas, to produce ion pairs. In the presence of an electric field the positive ions are attracted to the negative electrode, and the electrons to the positive electrode, thus causing an electric current to flow. As the applied voltage is increased, the ionisation current will increase from zero, until it reaches a constant value (Fig. 3.1); under these conditions all the ions are collected before recombination can occur, and saturation conditions have been reached. It is important that all ionisation chambers are operated under saturation conditions, when the ionisation current is proportional to the exposure rate. The current is measured using an electrometer. As the voltage is further increased, the ionisation current will again increase as gas multiplication takes place; that is, the initial ions are sufficiently accelerated to produce more ion pairs before they are collected. This is the region of the proportional counter. As the voltage is further increased, more gas multiplication takes place, and this is the region of the Geiger-Müller counter. Both the proportional counter and the Geiger-Müller counter are discussed in later sections.

In the ionisation chamber the electric charge, Q, produced by

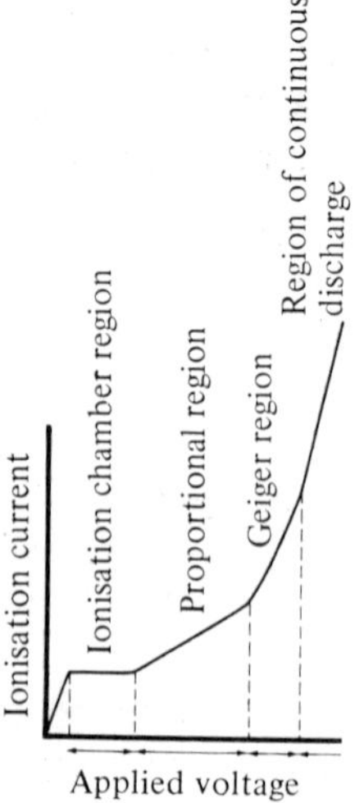

Fig. 3.1. Variation of ionisation current with applied voltage.

the passage of a single electron is equal to the product of the number of ion pairs formed, n, and the electronic charge, e, i.e.

$$Q = ne, \text{ where } e \text{ is equal to } 1.6 \times 10^{-19} \text{ coulombs (C)} \tag{3.1}$$

But the energy required to produce one ion pair is approximately 34 eV for energies between 0.08 MeV and 2 MeV. Therefore for an electron of energy 0.1 MeV,

$$n = \frac{0.1 \times 10^6}{34} = 3 \times 10^3 \text{ ion pairs}$$

and thus

$$Q = (3 \times 10^3)\,(1.6 \times 10^{-19})\text{C} = 5 \times 10^{-16}\,\text{C}$$

With a capacity of 100 picofarads (pf) the amplitude of the voltage pulse, V, due to a single β-particle of energy 0.1 MeV, would be given by

$$V = \frac{Q}{C} = \frac{5 \times 10^{-16}}{100 \times 10^{-12}} = 5 \times 10^{-6} \text{ volts (V), i.e. } 5 \text{ microvolts } (\mu\text{V})$$

Ionisation chambers may be used as pulse detectors, but require the use of highly stable, sensitive electronic equipment in order to detect these very small pulses, and are not used in this way for clinical work.

The electric current is equal to the number of ion pairs produced in unit time multiplied by the electronic charge, and is directly proportional to the intensity of the incident radiation and the volume of gas in the chamber. Ionisation currents, I, are usually measured by some form of electrometer or microammeter.

$$I = \frac{\mathrm{d}Q}{\mathrm{d}t} \tag{3.2}$$

$$= \frac{\mathrm{d}(ne)}{\mathrm{d}t} = \frac{e\,\mathrm{d}n}{\mathrm{d}t} \tag{3.3}$$

By definition, one roentgen (R) produces one electrostatic unit (e.s.u.) of charge in 0.001293 g of air (1 cm^3 air at NTP). Since the electronic charge is 4.8×10^{-10} e.s.u., the number of ion pairs produced is $1/(4.8 \times 10^{-10})$ per cm^3 air at NTP. Therefore the ionisation current which will be produced in an ionisation chamber of volume 100 cm^3, by an exposure rate of 1 R per minute can be calculated:

$$\frac{\mathrm{d}n}{\mathrm{d}t} = \frac{100}{(4.8 \times 10^{-10})60} \text{ ion pairs per second}$$

$$\therefore I = \frac{100(1.6 \times 10^{-19})}{(4.8 \times 10^{-10})60} \text{ C per second}$$

$$= 0.55 \times 10^{-9} \text{ amperes (A) for an exposure rate of 1 R per minute}$$

Expressed in SI units, the ionisation current produced by an exposure-rate in air of 1 C kg^{-1} per minute (which is equivalent to 3.88×10^3 R per minute: see Chapter 11) will be 2.13×10^{-6} A. The exposure-rate constants of commonly used radionuclides range from 0.1 to 18 R per hour (0.002 to 0.3 R per minute) per millicurie at 1 cm (0.0007 to 1.26 C kg^{-1} per hour per gigabecquerel); therefore in measuring quantities of radioactivity of the order of 100 μCi (3.7 MBq) up to 100 mCi (3.7 GBq) ionisation currents of the order of 10^{-13} up to 10^{-8} A will be obtained. In monitoring instruments which must be able to detect down to a fraction of the maximum permissible dose (approximately 3 mR per hour, or 0.05 mR per minute), the currents even with a larger chamber of 1000 cm^3 are only of the order of 10^{-14} A upward. The currents are generally measured by an electrometer, which measures the voltage difference across a load resistor. The ionisation current for a given exposure is dependent on the mass of air in the chamber, and therefore unless the chamber is hermetically sealed the current will vary with temperature and pressure. For unsealed chambers corrections for temperature and pressure must be made. The limit of sensitivity is due to the fact that in order to generate an adequate voltage signal, the load resistor must be very high; for example even if a 10^{12} ohm resistor is used the voltage signal with a current of 10^{-14} A will only be 10 mV. It is important that the insulation of the chamber electrodes is good so that the resistance of any possible leakage path is high compared with that of the load resistor. Cleanliness is obviously important in this context. The type of electrometer most commonly used is the MOSFET semiconductor device (metal oxide semiconductor field effect transistor) which will measure currents from 10^{-15} to 10^{-7} A. In the integrating dosemeter, which records total dose, the ionisation chamber is charged to a known value, and the total loss of charge over a known period of time is measured.

When ionisation chambers are used for assaying samples in units of radioactivity it is necessary to employ an instrument which has been calibrated with standardised samples, or to adopt a specified design of reference equipment for which calibration figures are available. This latter need was recognised by the National Physical Laboratory (NPL) in 1954 when prototype β and γ ionisation chambers were designed and tested for this purpose. The project was sponsored by the NPL Advisory Committee on Radioactive Standards and a limited number of β/γ ionisation chambers were produced in collaboration with the Atomic Energy Research Establishment, Harwell. Commercial models of the chamber, known as the type 1383A, became available during 1957. They were first manufactured by General Radiological Ltd, and subsequently by GEC-Elliott Automation Ltd.

Tests carried out at the NPL with standard γ-ray sources (^{24}Na, ^{60}Co, ^{131}I, ^{198}Au and ^{226}Ra) showed that over this energy range, chambers had the same calibration characteristics within about ±1%. Calibration figures published by the NPL for the 1383A chamber may be confidently applied to any chamber of this type provided that uniform measurement procedures are adopted. Assuming that the ionisation current is measured to an accuracy of ±1%, say, then the accuracy of standardisation of solutions relative to the published NPL calibration figures is about ±2%. The chamber is a combination of an unsealed re-entrant cylindrical chamber for γ-ray measurement and a 'parallel plate' chamber for β-ray measurements. Since the latter is little used in the clinical field, it will not be dealt with here, and Fig. 3.2 shows the re-entrant cylindrical chamber only. The inner and outer cylinders together with the circular base plate form one electrode which is at high potential. The intermediate cylinder is the collecting electrode which is at low potential, and insulated from the base plate; it is connected to the current measuring instrument, e.g. a DC amplifier or electrometer. The chamber has a brass liner to absorb β-radiation, and the original calibration figures were for use with this brass liner. A subsequent paper (Woods, 1970) gives a comprehensive list of calibration figures for the NPL γ-chamber used with and without liner. These are expressed in pA mCi^{-1} and range from 0.91 for chromium-51, through 4.7 for technetium-99m, up to 75.4 pA mCi^{-1} for sodium-24 (Table 3.1). The limit of measurement is governed by the background current which is about 0.01 pA; if the limiting current for accurate measurement is taken as 10 times background, this is 0.1 pA which corresponds to 0.1 mCi ^{51}Cr, 0.02 mCi ^{99m}Tc and 0.001 mCi ^{24}Na.

A similar instrument has been developed more recently by D.A. Pitman Ltd (Fig. 3.3) consisting basically of a re-entrant ionisation chamber and an electrometer. It is very useful for routine measurements of sample activity. The instrument is calibrated experimentally by the manufacturers for a large number of nuclides, and also for various sample volumes. When measuring a sample, the 'Isotope Factor' control is set to the calibration value, and the 'Sample Volume' control is set to the appropriate value; the digital meter will then display the total activity in millicuries. Corrections for temperature and pressure are applied by

Fig. 3.2. Standard ionisation chamber, type 1381A, showing re-entrant chamber only. (Modified from a drawing kindly supplied by The National Physical Laboratory, Division of Radiation Science and Acoustics.)

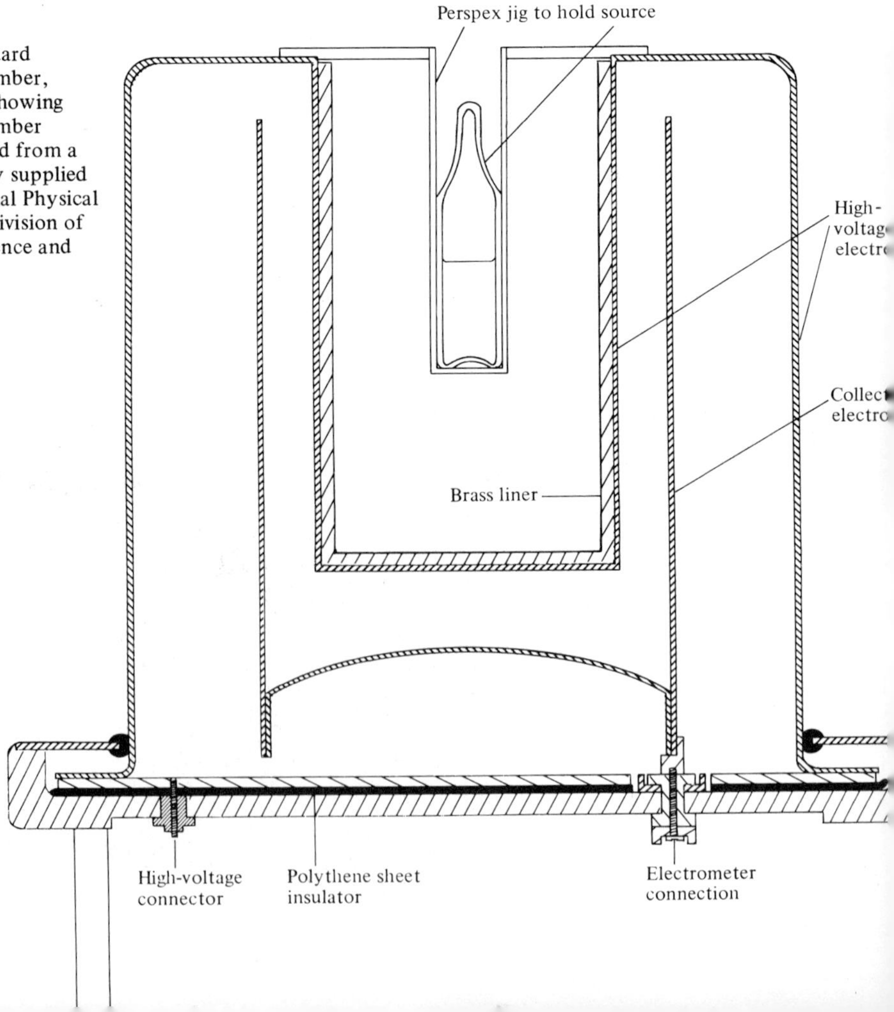

Table 3.1 *Mean values of ionisation currents (corrected to a pressure of 760 mm Hg and a temperature of 22 °C in chamber type 1383 A, serial number 14)*

Radioactive nuclide	With liner (pA mCi^{-1})	Without liner (pA mCi^{-1})	Standard error of the mean (%)	Random error (%)	Systematic error (%)
^{22}Na	50.6	54.8	±0.08	±0.3	±1
^{24}Na	75.4	84.2	±0.15	±0.4	±1
^{42}K	6.04	82.1	±0.2	±0.7	±1
^{46}Sc	44.8	48.0	±0.1	±0.3	±1
^{51}Cr	0.91	1.05	±0.35	±1.0	±1.5
^{54}Mn	19.4	21.0	±0.15	±0.5	±1
^{56}Mn	35.1	51.9	±0.1	±0.3	±0.4
^{57}Co	4.35	11.1	±0.2	±0.9	±2
^{59}Fe	25.4	27.4	±0.14	±0.6	±1
^{60}Co	52.9	56.7	±0.08	±0.3	±0.5
^{75}Se	–	18.81	±0.3	±0.8	±4
^{82}Br	61.4	66.6	±0.14	±1.4	±3
^{85}Sr	13.05	14.36	±0.07	±0.2	±2
^{87m}Sr	–	9.77	±0.2	±0.6	±2
^{95}Nb	18.09	19.55	±0.03	±0.1	±1
^{99m}Tc	4.7	9.6	±0.35	±2	±3
^{113m}In	–	8.44	±0.08	±0.3	±2
^{131}I	10.35	12.27	±0.1	±0.5	±3
^{132}I	–	58.0	±0.25	±0.7	±2
^{137}Cs	13.7	15.4	±0.25	±0.7	±5
^{139}Ce	4.71	12.68	±0.2	±0.5	±1.5
^{141}Ce	2.641	6.144	±0.1	±0.3	±1.5
^{198}Au	10.79	12.45	±0.1	±0.3	±1.0
^{203}Hg	6.92	9.83	±0.1	±0.3	±3

Reproduced from *Int. J. Appl. Radiat. Isot.* (1970), **21**, 752–3, by kind permission of the National Physical Laboratory.
These values apply to 1 g of solution in an NPL type 2 ml ampoule.

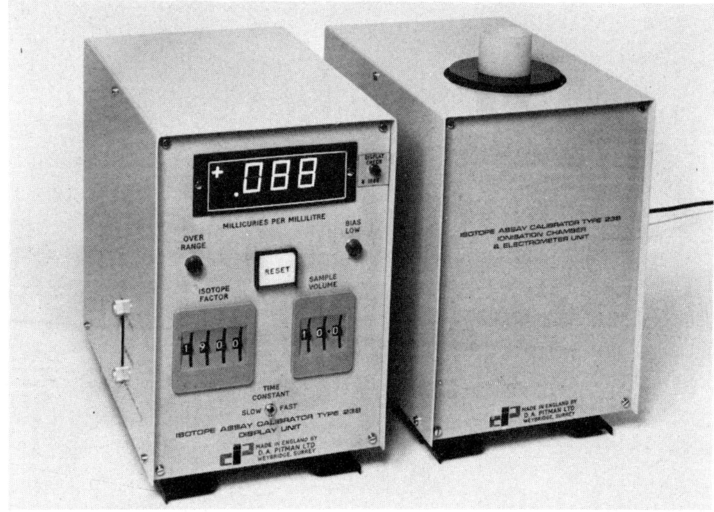

Fig. 3.3. Isotope assay calibrator. (Photograph kindly supplied by D.A. Pitman Ltd.)

adjusting a 'Calibration' control. As with the 1383A chamber it is important that the applied voltage is maintained at the correct level, so that saturation conditions apply, and that regular measurements are made on a standard radioactive source in order to check consistency of performance. The manufacturer's calibration figures should be checked against reference equipment before the chamber is put into clinical use.

Both instruments described above require pressure and temperature corrections to be made and in addition the 1383A chamber has a large geometry dependence. Other commercial systems are available with sealed chambers but only the 1383A has the advantage of direct traceability to a national standardising laboratory.

To overcome the limitations of existing systems the NPL in 1974 proposed a scheme based on two classes of instrument. The class I (secondary standard) system would incorporate a high-pressure graphite electrode ionisation chamber with a smooth (monotonic) energy response. The class II (field) system would also be a sealed chamber but of simpler construction. The NPL would then in future provide calibration figures for both ionisation chambers as had previously been done for the 1383A, and in addition an energy response curve for the class I chamber. The class I chamber could then be used to standardise virtually any radionuclide, provided its decay scheme details were known. The new class II chamber would have an enhanced sensitivity at low energies relative to the 1383A, could be used for quite large vessels and would have an automatic readout system in units of activity. The intention of the NPL proposal was that Regional Centres in the UK Health Service would hold a class I system and other users would need only a class II system. However the Department of Health has decided to support production of the class II system only. The response of all class II chambers will be traceable to NPL, and Regional Centres will be provided with specially calibrated systems. With the original proposal it would have been possible for Regional Centres to standardise any new radionuclide, whereas with the present proposal the required calibration figures will need to be provided by NPL. The prototype of the class II chamber is under construction and it is hoped that this system will soon be available commercially.

Ionisation chambers are also used for monitoring purposes, for measuring exposure rates. Any ionisation chamber will have a certain energy dependence, that is for a constant exposure rate the response may be different for γ-rays of different energy. This effect is not of great importance when measuring quantities of radioactivity since the response is calibrated for different energies. However, with a radiation monitor the response is required to be independent of energy; this is partly achieved by making the wall of the chamber of air-equivalent material and building up the wall thickness for high-energy radiations to effect electronic equilibrium. Portable instruments are used in surveys of radiation levels, their sensitivity depending on the size of the chamber and the lower limit of current measurement. A typical instrument is shown in Fig. 3.4(*a*). The detector is an unsealed air ionisation

Fig. 3.4. (*a*) Portable γ-radiation monitor. (*b*) Energy response curve. (Kindly supplied by Alrad Instruments Ltd.)

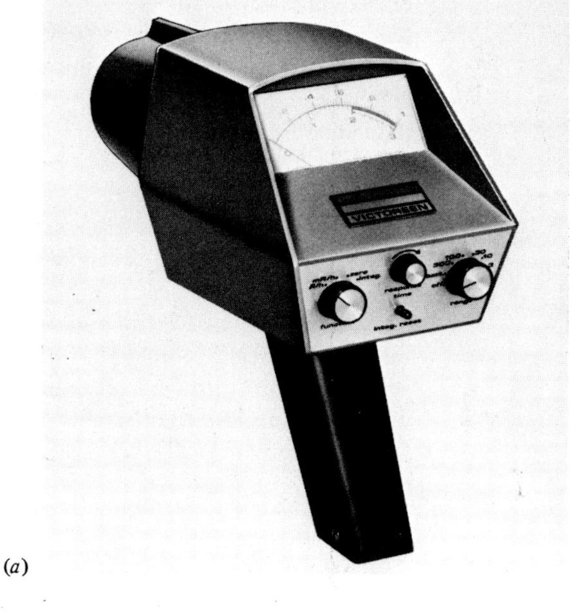

(*a*)

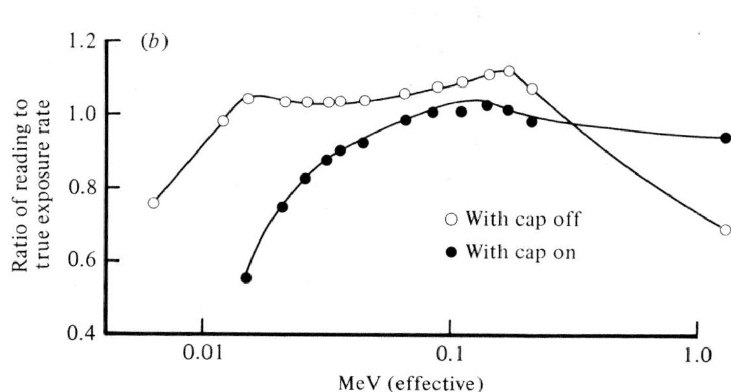

chamber, made with walls of expanded polystyrene, with a volume of 275 cc, and a readout meter calibrated in ranges from 3 mR per hour to 1000R per hour. The energy response curve is shown in Fig. 3.4(*b*), and is seen to be fairly constant between 0.03 MeV and 0.2 MeV without the cap; for higher energies the use of the equilibrium cap maintains the response approximately constant, although 5–10% lower than the reading without the cap, up to 1 MeV.

Pulse detectors

Proportional counters

The basic principle of the proportional counter is the same as that of the ionisation chamber, except that a very high voltage gradient exists in the vicinity of the positive electrode. Because of this, each electron produced by an initial ionising event undergoes a high acceleration and is capable of further ionisation. Gas multiplication of up to one-thousand is possible, and produces a pulse of 0.1 to 10 mV, but still strictly proportional to the energy of the initial electron. Pulses of this size are more readily detectable than the microvolt pulses from an ionisation chamber. Proportional counters are either windowless or have very thin windows, and are used for measurement of solid sources of β-emitting nuclides. They are usually filled with argon/methane mixtures or pure methane, and are operated at atmospheric pressure, the gas being allowed to flow through the côunter at a rate sufficient to prevent diffusion of air into the chamber. Proportional counters are not widely used in medical work, and will not therefore be considered in detail.

Fig. 3.5. Geiger counter: (*a*) photograph and (*b*) drawing.

(*a*)

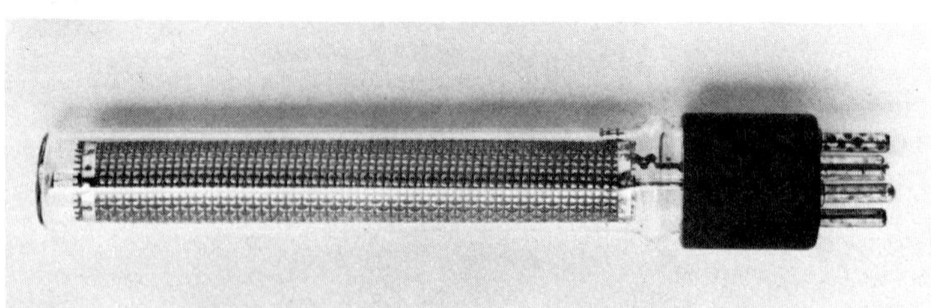

(*b*)

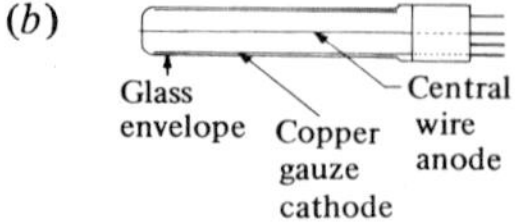

Geiger–Müller tubes

The Geiger–Müller counter is essentially an ionisation chamber operated at such a high voltage that the gas multiplication becomes an avalanche of electrons, and a large pulse of the order of 1 V may be obtained. The detailed mechanism is complex, and a good description is given by Faires & Parks (1973, pp. 131–8).

The normal construction of the counter is a cylindrical outer cathode and a central wire anode sealed into a glass tube which is filled with a gas or mixture of gases (Fig. 3.5). The main constituent of the gas mixture is a readily ionised gas, usually a mixture of two or more of the inert or rare gases, helium, argon or neon. There is also a small amount of a halogen gas which acts as a quenching agent to prevent a discharge being re-initiated when the positive ions reach the cathode.

Although the collection time of the electrons in a Geiger counter is fast, less than 1 microsecond, the slow movement of the positive ions renders the counter inoperative for a period of time after the initiation of the ionising event. A further period of time elapses before the counter is capable of registering a further pulse; this time was originally known as 'resolution time' but will be referred to here as dead-time, to conform with the definition used in scintillation counting.

Because of the large sizes of the pulses the accessory electronic equipment is relatively simple; it is shown schematically in Fig. 3.6. Basically it comprises the high-voltage unit which supplies the voltage across the counter, a low-voltage supply to supply power to the other units, a quenching probe unit or cathode follower incorporating low-gain amplification, and a scaling unit, or scaler–timer unit. The probe unit is used to apply electronically an accurately known 'paralysis time' which is longer than the dead-time, and using this value it is possible to apply a correction for count losses which occur at higher count-rates (equation 4.1, p. 42).

Although the Geiger counter has the advantage of simplicity it has several disadvantages. It is relatively inefficient, the amplitude

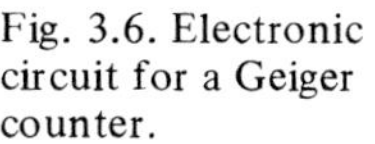
Fig. 3.6. Electronic circuit for a Geiger counter.

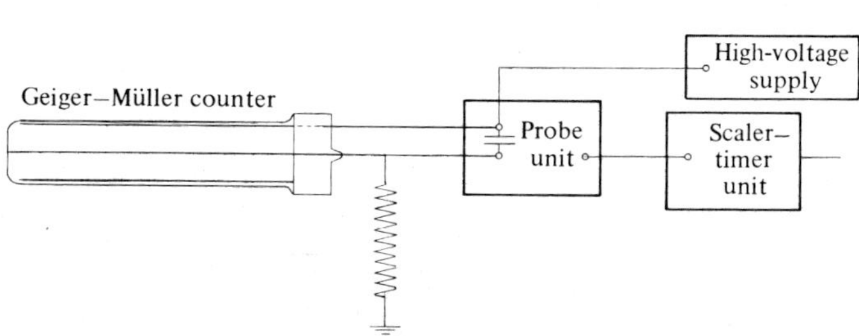

of the output pulse is not proportional to the energy of the electron initiating the event as in the proportional counter, and it has a long dead-time. It has been largely superseded by scintillation detectors except in the measurement of solid samples of low-energy β-emitters, and in monitoring instruments for detection of low-energy β-emitters such as carbon-14.

In operation, the value of the applied voltage is quite critical. As the voltage is increased no pulses are registered until a certain voltage is reached, when the count-rate increases rapidly until the threshold voltage, then remains approximately constant for 150 to 200 V, after which it increases again (Fig. 3.7). The flat region of the curve is referred to as the plateau; the threshold voltage, and the slope and length of the plateau are quoted by the manufacturer for each counter. The slope should be not greater than 0.5% per volt, and the counter should be operated at the mid-point of the plateau, usually about 100 V above threshold voltage.

Scintillation counters

Scintillation counters are at present the most widely used type of detector. Scintillators are materials in which the absorption of β-rays, or secondary electrons produced by γ-ray interaction, produces luminescence as well as ionisation. A scintillation detector consists essentially of a scintillator which produces light quanta, and a photomultiplier tube which converts the light quanta into output electrical pulses which appear at its anode (Fig. 3.8). Associated electronic equipment is used to select and count pulses of appropriate amplitude. An important feature of scintillation detectors is that proportionality is maintained between the energy of the incident γ-ray photon and the amplitude of those output

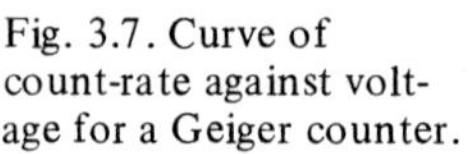

Fig. 3.7. Curve of count-rate against voltage for a Geiger counter.

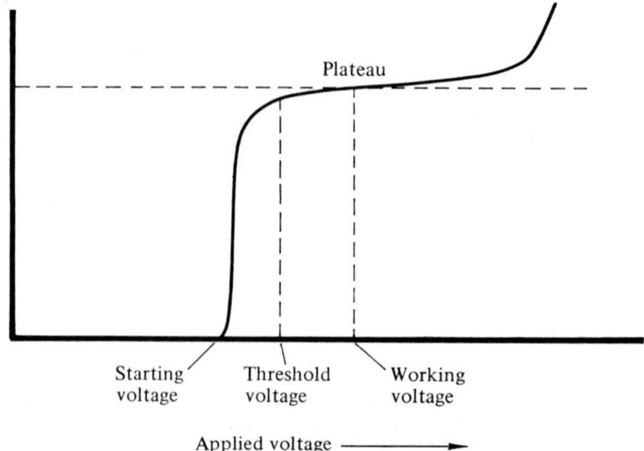

pulses which represent the photopeak. This is considered in more detail below.

There are three main types of scintillators: sodium iodide, organic solid and organic liquid. Each has specific properties which render it suitable for different applications and which affect the electronic circuitry. They will therefore be dealt with separately. However, all of them use a photomultiplier tube to convert light quanta into electrical pulses, and it is therefore appropriate to describe this first.

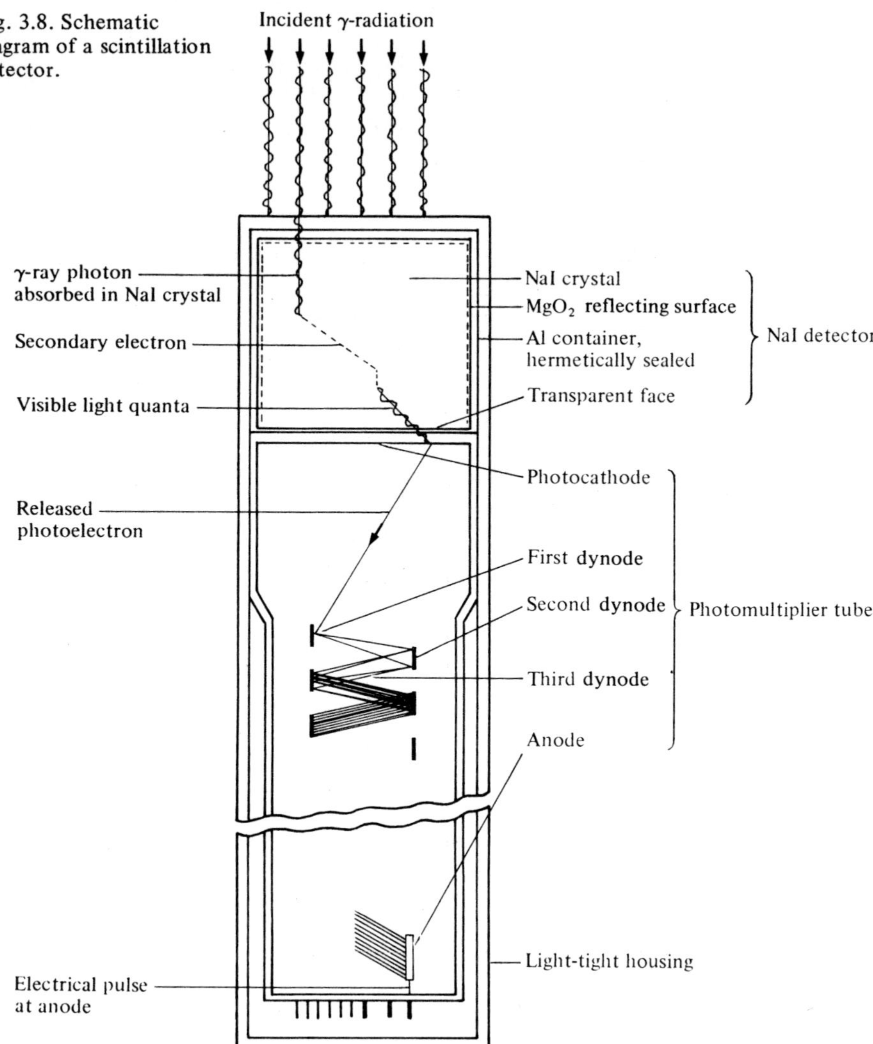

Fig. 3.8. Schematic diagram of a scintillation detector.

Photomultiplier (PM) tubes. A PM tube (Fig. 3.9) is a device which converts light energy into electrical energy. It consists essentially of an evacuated glass envelope containing a photosensitive cathode, several electrodes called dynodes, and a collecting anode. The mode of operation is shown in Fig. 3.8. Light photons incident on the photocathode give rise to the emission of photoelectrons. By means of a resistor chain, across which is applied a high voltage of the order of 1000 V, a voltage difference is established between each successive pair of dynodes (Fig. 3.9*b*).

Fig. 3.9. (*a*) Photograph of a PM tube. (*b*) Diagram of PM tube and connections.

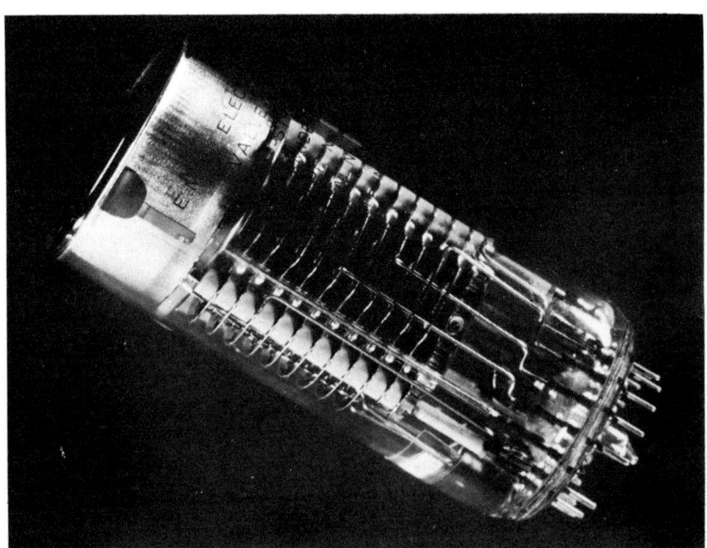

(*a*)

Photocathode
Resistor chain
High-voltage supply
Dynodes
Anode

(*b*)

This causes each photoelectron to be accelerated across the first dynode stage, and it acquires enough energy to eject several electrons; the process is repeated for each stage and electron multiplication takes place.

If an electron of energy E produces m_1 quanta of visible light in the scintillator, and the optical efficiency is such that a fraction m_2 of these reach the photocathode of the PM tube, which has a quantum efficiency of m_3, then the number of photoelectrons released at the photocathode will be $m_1\ m_2\ m_3$. With a multiplication factor of R for each of the n dynode stages, the number of electrons collected at the anode will be $m_1\ m_2\ m_3\ R^n$. The charge Q collected at the anode is given by

$$Q = m_1 m_2 m_3\ R^n e\ \mathrm{C} \tag{3.4}$$

where e is the electronic charge (1.6×10^{-19} C). Typical values for a 0.1 MeV electron are:

$$m_1 = 10^3$$

$$m_2 = 0.5$$

$$m_3 = 0.15$$

$$m_1 m_2 m_3 = 75$$

$$\left.\begin{matrix} R = 4.5 \\ n = 10 \end{matrix}\right\} R^n = 3.5 \times 10^6$$

Substituting these values in equation 3.4, $Q = 42 \times 10^{-12}$ C for a 0.1 MeV electron.

A typical sensitivity for a charge-sensitive amplifier is 20 to 100 mV output for 10^{-12} C of charge from the PM output, giving pulses of 0.84–4.2 V for 0.1 MeV electrons. For one electron liberated at the photocathode the value of Q will be 0.56×10^{-12} C; the background noise is therefore 10 to 50 mV and this is the limiting factor in the sensitivity of the scintillation counter to low-energy radiation.

The overall gain and therefore the stability of the system is dependent on the luminescent properties of the scintillator, on the optical efficiency of the scintillator–PM coupling, on the PM gain (which is also dependent on the stability of the high-voltage supply and of the resistor chain), and also on the amplifier gain.

Sodium iodide detectors. Sodium iodide (NaI) crystals, activated with thallium, are widely used for the detection of γ-rays because of their high sensitivity and relatively good energy resolution. As pointed out in the beginning of this chapter, for a γ-ray to be detected it must be absorbed, with the production of secondary electrons. The high sensitivity of NaI detectors compared with, for example, ionisation chambers or Geiger counters is due to their high density compared with that of air (3.67 g cm^{-3} against 0.001293 g cm^{-3}), and the higher atomic number of iodine (Z = 53). These factors combine to give NaI a higher linear absorption coefficient. The intrinsic counting efficiency of a scintillator for γ-rays can be obtained by calculating the fraction of γ-rays which it absorbs. It will obviously depend on the relative geometrical configuration of the source and crystal, and the energy of the γ-radiation, as well as the density and atomic number of the scintillator.

The good energy resolution of the NaI detector is due to its high atomic number, and the consequent large photoelectric component. The number of light quanta produced by any one electron is proportional to its energy loss in the scintillator. As will be shown in Chapter 11, in photoelectric absorption the whole of the energy of the incident γ-ray photon is given to the secondary electron. If, in addition, that secondary electron is wholly absorbed in the scintillator, then the number of visible light quanta produced (m_1 of equation 3.4) will be proportional to the energy of the incident γ-ray photon. It follows from equation 3.4 that the amplitude of the PM output pulses will also be proportional to the energy of the incident γ-ray photon. It is also evident that those photoelectrons which are not wholly absorbed

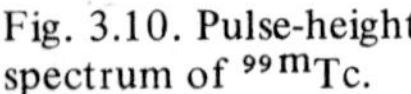
Fig. 3.10. Pulse-height spectrum of ^{99m}Tc.

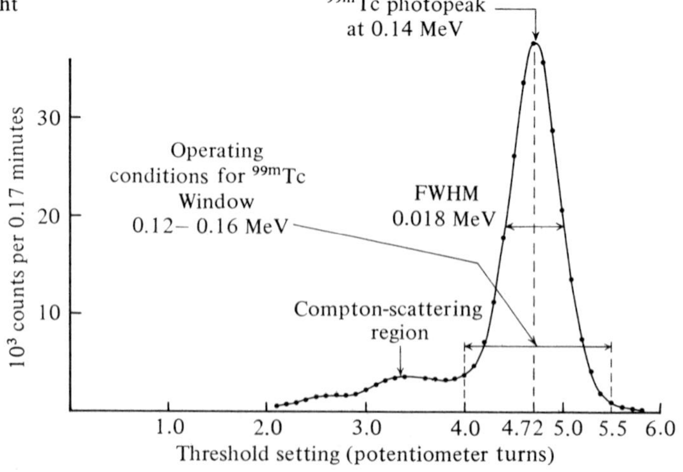

in the crystal will produce output pulses of lower energy, as will also the Compton electrons (see Chapter 11, p. 192) whether or not they are wholly absorbed in the crystal. Therefore for a mono-energetic beam of γ-radiation incident on a NaI crystal the distribution of amplitudes of the output pulses will show a main photopeak, and also a broader scatter band. The pulse-height spectrum for ^{99m}Tc as obtained with a 3-inch diameter, 3-inch thick NaI well-shaped crystal is shown in Fig. 3.10. The main γ-ray energy of ^{99m}Tc is 0.14 MeV, which occurs in 98.6% disintegrations. The photopeak corresponding to the pulses obtained when the γ-rays are absorbed by the photoelectric effect, is clearly seen. The flatter low-energy part of the curve corresponds to γ-rays absorbed by Compton scattering. It is usual to operate scintillation counters to detect pulses in the photopeak only, thereby reducing the background counts and also the effect of scattered radiation.

The energy resolution of a detector is defined as the full-width-at-half-maximum (FWHM) of the photopeak, and is often expressed as a percentage of the energy of the photopeak. In Fig. 3.10 the 0.14 MeV peak occurs at a potentiometer setting of 4.72 and has a count-rate of 37 000 counts for 0.17 minutes. Half-maximum is, therefore, 18 500 counts per 0.17 minutes, and the width of the photopeak at this counting-rate is 0.6 turns and corresponds to 0.018 MeV; the energy resolution is 13%. The operating conditions for ^{99m}Tc used for sample counting are a threshold of 0.12 MeV and a window of 0.04 MeV, i.e. 32%. In a system with good energy resolution it is possible to use dual-

Fig. 3.11. Pulse-height spectrum of ^{51}Cr and ^{125}I.

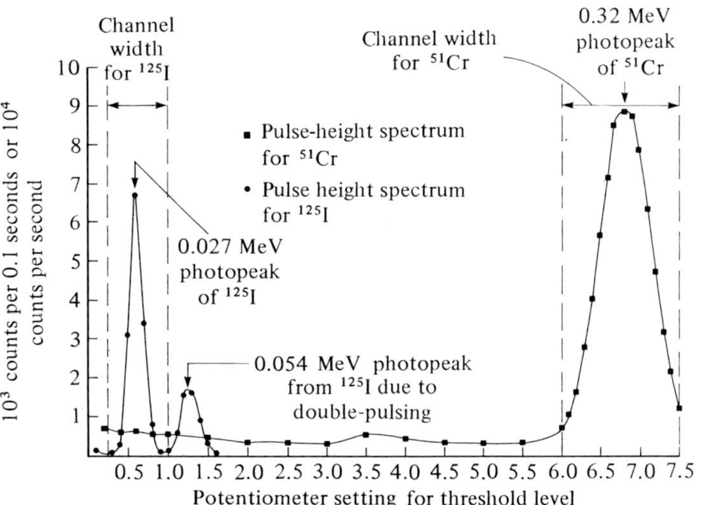

nuclide techniques, that is it is possible to measure simultaneously the activity of two radionuclides present in one source. The principle of this is shown in Fig. 3.11 which shows on the same curve the pulse-height spectra for ^{51}Cr and ^{125}I. In a scintillation system with two pulse-height analysers, counts can be made simultaneously in two channels as shown, corresponding to the ^{51}Cr and the ^{125}I photopeaks. The counts in the higher-energy channel will be due to ^{51}Cr alone, while the counts in the lower-energy channel will be due to the ^{125}I but also to part of the Compton scattering of the ^{51}Cr. A correction can be applied by counting a pure ^{51}Cr standard source in both channels and calculating the ratio of ^{51}Cr counts in the two channels.

NaI detectors are almost universally used for counting liquid or solid samples of γ-emitting radionuclides. They are also used for measurements on patients, but the equipment is specialised and will be considered separately in Chapter 7.

There is a wide variety of NaI crystals which are commercially available. Their manufacture is a skilled procedure, and a high standard is required. Firstly, it is essential that the optical quality of the crystal is good, in order that it is transparent to the wavelength of light emitted. Secondly, it must be hermetically sealed because NaI is deliquescent and a crystal rapidly deteriorates when exposed to air. The crystals are usually cylindrical or well-shaped, and are housed in an aluminium casing with a glass face which is optically coupled to the photocathode of the PM tube. The crystal and PM tube are often manufactured in one integral assembly.

For counting samples of small volume, re-entrant or well-shaped crystals are used. These have the advantage of high sensitivity which is not very dependent on the shape and volume of the sample. For counting samples of large volume, one or two cylindrical detectors are used in a fixed geometrical relationship with respect to the sample.

The optimum size of crystal, and also the thickness of the front face of the container, is dependent on the energy of the radiation to be detected. Low-energy γ-radiation and β-radiation will be readily absorbed in a thin crystal, but high-energy γ-radiation needs a thick crystal. The intrinsic efficiency of a cylindrical NaI crystal of thickness x for a parallel beam of γ-rays of energy E is equal to the percentage of γ-rays 'absorbed' in the crystal. (This assumes that counts over the whole energy spectrum are accepted.) It may be calculated as follows:

$I = I_0 e^{-\mu_E x}$ (equation 11.3, p. 191)

γ-rays 'absorbed' $= I_0 - I = I_0\ (1 - e^{-\mu_E x})$

where I_0 = intensity of incident radiation

I = intensity of emergent radiation

μ_E = linear attenuation coefficient for NaI for γ-rays of energy E

x = thickness of the NaI crystal

The percentage 'absorption', ϵ, is calculated by

$$\epsilon = \frac{(I_0 - I)}{I_0}\ 100 = (1 - e^{-\mu_E x})\ 100 \qquad (3.5)$$

Values of ϵ for different energies, for NaI crystals of thicknesses from 0.64 cm to 10.16 cm are given in Table 3.2. When the counter is operated to count only the photopeak the efficiency will be lower because only a fraction of the γ-rays absorbed will give rise to pulses in the photopeak. Values of the photopeak efficiency for well-shaped crystals of two sizes are given in Table 3.3. The thickness of the aluminium housing is usually of the order of 1 mm, but for the detection of low-energy γ-emitters such as ^{125}I, and of β-emitters, a beryllium window is sometimes used.

The basic circuitry for a manual sample counter is shown in Fig. 3.12 and comprises high-voltage supply, low-voltage supply, pre-amplifier, amplifier and pulse-height analyser, and scaler–

Table 3.2 *Calculated intrinsic efficiencies for NaI crystals for a parallel beam of γ-rays*

γ-ray energy (MeV)	Thickness of NaI crystals in cm (and inches)					
	0.64 (¼)	1.27 (½)	2.54 (1)	5.08 (2)	7.62 (3)	10.16 (4)
0.122	96	100	100	100	100	100
0.140	94	100	100	100	100	100
0.279	45	71	79	96	100	100
0.364	34	56	68	90	97	100
0.412	30	51	64	87	95	98
0.511	26	45	57	81	92	96
0.622	21	38	50	75	87	94
0.840	19	35	45	70	83	91
1.17	16	30	40	63	78	86
1.33	15	28	37	60	75	84
2.62	12	23	30	51	65	75
2.75	11	22	29	50	64	69

timer unit. The high-voltage supply is needed to maintain the potential across the PM tube, and since the gain is very dependent on that voltage, it is necessary to have a highly stabilised supply. It is also necessary to be able to set the high voltage to the required value, and a fine resettable adjustment is essential. Most high-voltage supply units have outputs which are continuously variable between, for example, 300 V and 1500 V, with a helipot control so that they can be reset to within 1 V. A typical specification of stability is 0.01% for a 10% change in mains voltage or for a 1 deg C temperature variation.

The function of the pre-amplifier is mainly that of impedance matching between the detector and main amplifier. Scintillation detectors are, as are all radiation transducers, low-capacitance high-impedance devices, therefore the capacitance of the output cable from detector to amplifier is liable to attenuate the output pulse. A short, low-capacitance cable and a pre-amplifier placed near the detector will minimise this effect and can be designed to give a low-impedance output so that long cables can be used to the amplifier. The simplest type of pre-amplifier is a cathode follower, or emitter follower, and one often used to be incorporated in the detector head, necessitating low-voltage power supply

Table 3.3 *Percentage photopeak efficiencies for 1 ml samples in NaI well-shaped crystals*

γ-ray energy (MeV)	Size of NaI crystal	
	4.44 cm diam. × 5.08 cm high[a] (1¼ in × 2 in)	7.62 cm diam. × 7.62 cm high[b] (3 in × 3 in)
0.080	97	95
0.142	88	96
0.279	49	69.5
0.321	36	58.5
0.364	31	50
0.411	24	45
0.511	17.5	36
0.662	11.5	25
0.835	9.4	21.5
0.885	8.4	17
1.11	6.7	16.5
1.17	6.0	15
1.27	5.5	14
1.33	5.3	13
2.75	2.5	7.5

[a] Size of well: 2.9 cm diam. × 3.8 cm deep (¾ in × 1½ in).
[b] Size of well: 2.54 cm diam. × 5.08 cm deep (1 in × 2 in).

to the head. More recently a charge-sensitive pre-amplifier has been used. This type has the great advantage over voltage-sensitive pre-amplifiers that the amplitude of the output voltage is independent of the detector capacitance and of stray capacitance.

The pulse-height analyser (PHA), as its name implies, is used to look at the frequency distribution of pulse amplitude, and to select the part of the spectrum to be used for counting. It may take the form of a simple discriminator which merely cuts out any pulses below a pre-set threshold, or it may have an upper cut-off also, so that only pulses within a pre-set range of amplitude are transmitted for counting. This range is usually referred to as window or channel width. The analyser has two potentiometer settings: one which controls the lower cut-off referred to as the discriminator, threshold, or lower-level control, and the other which sets the channel width. The pulse-height spectrum is obtained by setting the window to a very narrow width and obtaining counts as the threshold is set to different values, starting at the minimum and increasing to cover the whole range of pulse amplitudes present. The output pulses from the PHA are of a standard shape and amplitude, and are fed to the input of a scaling unit, or ratemeter, which counts the pulses. Although in the simplest of systems the scaler can be operated manually, and the time of counting recorded with a stop-watch, most scalers are operated in conjunction with a timing unit which automatically triggers the scaling unit to start counting and measures the counting time. There is usually provision in such a scaler–timer unit for

Fig. 3.12. Electronic circuit for scintillation detector.

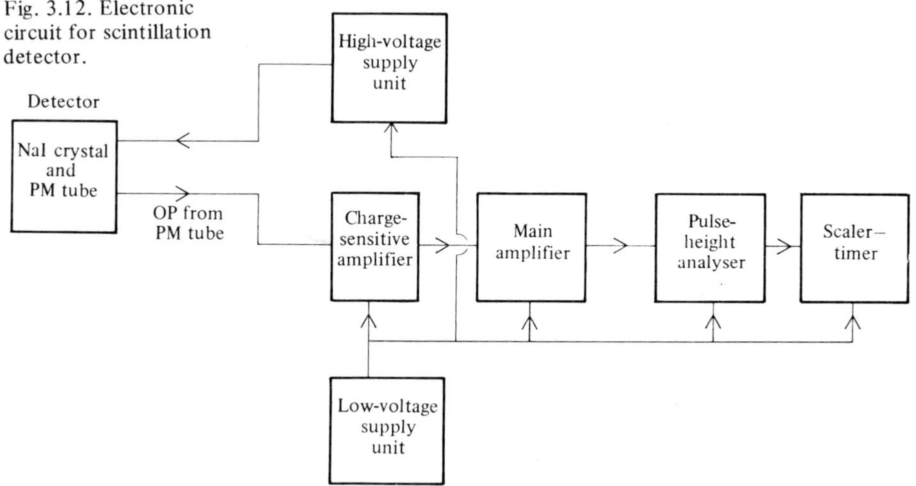

pre-setting either the time or the total counts required. Most scaling units have provision for operating a recording instrument such as a printer. Ratemeters record count-rates and are useful for quick measurements, when accuracy is not of great importance. The input pulses charge up a capacitor (C) which leaks away across a resistor (R); the potential across the resistor, which is proportional to the rate of arrival of pulses, is read by a high-impedance voltmeter calibrated in pulses per second. The time constant, T, is equal to CR, and a time of at least 2.3 T should be allowed before taking the reading, which will then have risen to 90% of its steady reading. The output from a ratemeter may be used to operate a chart recorder.

There are now many sophisticated automatic sample changers available. These can be loaded with large numbers of samples, up to 500, which they then place in succession in the NaI well-shaped detector, for counting, and automatically record the results. The basic electronics is the same as in the above system, but in addition there is a controlling system which moves the first sample into position for counting, senses when it is ready, starts the timer–scaler, senses when counting stops, initiates the transfer back to the tray of samples, and the printing-out of the result, senses when the sample is back in the tray, moves the sample-tray forward, and initiates the cycle all over again. With some systems it is possible to program for different batches to be counted with different settings of the PHA, so that, for example, 20 samples can be counted for ^{51}Cr and ^{125}I, another 20 samples for ^{131}I only, etc. The results may be printed out by a typewriter or punched out on to paper tape for computer processing.

Organic scintillator detectors. There are two types of organic scintillators: liquid and solid. They differ from NaI in several respects. Because of their low atomic number, the proportion of incident γ-rays which are totally absorbed is much smaller, and therefore the energy spectrum contains more Compton scattering than photoelectric peak. Consequently energy resolution is poor. The efficiency with which electron energy is converted to light energy is also much lower. Referring to the calculation for the voltage amplitude of the pulse (equation 3.4 *et seq.*), it will be seen that this will be appreciably smaller, and not so well separated from the background. Organic scintillators have one advantage – that of being faster, because of the short duration of the scintillation. Solid organic scintillators are not very much used, because of the disadvantages described, except where very large volume detectors are required. The basic electronics is the same as that for NaI detectors except that greater amplification is needed, and that a simple discriminator is adequate because there is no well-defined photopeak.

Liquid scintillation detectors. These are widely used for counting low-energy β-emitters. The main problem with these is that the β-radiation is of such short range that it is absorbed in the sample itself before it reaches the surface. To overcome this problem the radioactive sample is added directly into the liquid scintillator; it is therefore in immediate contact with the scintillator and can be counted with 100% geometrical efficiency and without any self-absorption losses. Liquid scintillators must be compatible with the radioactive samples to be counted. There are many commercially available. They consist of solvent and solute. The solvent is usually toluene or p-dioxane, the latter having the advantage of being miscible with water, which is useful for incorporating body fluids. The solute is the scintillator, which converts the excitation energy absorbed in the solvent to visible light quanta; a commonly used solute is 2,5-diphenyloxazole, known as PPO, with a small addition of 1,4-*bis*-2-(5-phenyloxazoly)-benzene, known as POPOP. The preparation of a sample consists of adding the radioactive sample, usually containing tritium (hydrogen-3) or carbon-14, to the standard volume, usually 5 ml, of the liquid scintillator. It is important that the addition of the sample should not affect the scintillation process. Such interference is referred to as a quenching effect, and there are two known effects – chemical quenching, which causes loss of emission of light, and optical quenching, which causes loss of transmission of light – both of which give rise to reduced efficiency. In relative measurements it is important to ensure that all samples are identical with respect to chemical content and physical properties. If this is not possible it is necessary to apply quenching corrections, and there are three ways of doing this (Belcher, 1971).

The limit of detection using a scintillation counter is, as was seen early in this chapter, dependent on the relative sizes of scintillator pulse and PM noise. A good liquid scintillator gives about seven photons per keV of β-ray energy, which, with the 5.6 keV β-radiation of tritium, gives about 40 photons. Referring to equation 3.4, it will be seen that even if all the light photons reach the photocathode (i.e. $m_2 = 1$) the number of photoelectrons released will only be about six, which means that the signal will not be much above the noise due to thermionic emission by the photocathode. The first liquid scintillation detectors were operated at low temperature, using liquid nitrogen for cooling, in order to reduce the background. The associated electronics was very similar to that for NaI detectors except that greater amplification was necessary. Now coincidence circuits are used; a second photomultiplier is added and an event is only recorded if it produces coincident pulses at the anode of both PM tubes. In this way the background noise is eliminated. As with the NaI detectors, many sophisticated automatic sample-changers are available.

The main practical problem is the preparation of the sample so that it will not interfere with the properties of the scintillator, and the appropriate skills and techniques have to be acquired in this specialised field.

Solid-state detectors

These are the latest type of detector to find useful applications, but are not yet widely used in medical work. Their main advantages are good linear response with energy, excellent energy resolution and fast response; their main disadvantage is low γ-ray sensitivity.

Semiconductor radiation detectors are made of single crystals of high-purity silicon and germanium; there are two main types, the diffused p–n junction and the lithium-drifted p–i–n structure. Such detectors are often referred to as solid-state detectors because the crystals act effectively as a solid-state version of a gas ionisation chamber. Whereas in the latter the passage of a charged particle, e.g. β-particle, produces ion pairs, in the solid-state detector electron-hole pairs are formed. Since the energy required to create an electron-hole pair is only 3.5 eV for silicon and 2.94 eV for germanium, compared with 33.7 eV required to produce an ion pair, approximately 10 times as much charge is collected for the same energy β-particle. Thus the pulses are much larger, and this is why the energy resolution is so much better.

For an electron of energy 0.1 MeV

$$Q = ne$$

$$n = \frac{0.1 \times 10^6}{3.5} = 3 \times 10^4 \text{ electron-hole pairs}$$

$$Q = (3 \times 10^4)(1.6 \times 10^{-19})\text{ C}$$

$$= 5 \times 10^{-15}\text{ C}$$

With a counter capacitance, C, of 10 pf per unit area, the output voltage, V, for a 1 cm^2 detector is given by

$$V = \frac{Q}{C} = \frac{5 \times 10^{-15}}{10 \times 10^{-12}} = 0.5 \text{ mV}$$

This compares with 5 μV for a gas ionisation chamber.

The main use of solid-state detectors is in γ-ray spectroscopy, where sensitivity is not important, and in dosimetry.

The lower limit of detection for γ-radiation is about 1 millirad (mrad) per minute, which is 20 times the maximum permissible level, and the upper limit 5000 rad per minute. These detectors are therefore most useful in measurement of high dose-rates, or where they can be used as integrating dosemeters.

References

Belcher, E.H. (1971). Measurements of radioactivity *in vitro.* In *Radioisotopes in Medical Diagnosis*, ed. E.H. Belcher & H. Vetter, pp. 97–100. London: Butterworth.

Faires, R.A. & Parks, B.H. (1973). Geiger–Müller counter. In *Radioisotope Laboratory Techniques*, pp. 131–8. London: Butterworth.

Woods, M.J. (1970). Calibration figures for the type 1383A ionisation chamber. *Int. J. Appl. Radiat. Isot.* **21** 752–3.

4. Radioactivity measurements on samples, and statistics

Quality control on equipment

The first step in achieving good results is to ensure that the equipment is operated under optimum conditions, and that it is reliable in performance. At the time of its installation measurements must be made to establish optimum operating conditions, and checks carried out to ensure that the performance is up to the required specification. There should then be a definite schedule for weekly and daily checks, and the results of these must be carefully recorded. A regular examination of these records may reveal a trend, or variations outside the statistical limit, which points to an incipient or intermittent fault at an early stage, before it is evident in the results. Regular inspection and maintenance should be carried out by a competent service engineer and a log-book kept of these checks, and of any faults which arise in the equipment.

Ionisation chambers

As shown in Chapter 3, it is essential that ionisation chambers are operated under saturation conditions. The manufacturers normally specify the voltage required to achieve saturation over the complete range of the instrument, and incorporate a meter to read the voltage across the electrodes. This must always be checked before use. When setting up a new instrument, checks should be made for linearity of response over the whole range. Ionisation chamber instruments for measuring quantities of radioactivity should be calibrated directly, or indirectly via a standard reference chamber, using standard sources of radionuclides with radiation energies covering the range of energies to be used. Such standard sources are obtainable from the National Physical Laboratory and the Radiochemical Centre. For most isotope assay calibrators the manufacturers will give calibration factors, but these should be checked. The accuracy of radiation-exposure measuring instruments is not quite so critical, but these should also be checked with known exposure-rates. Daily checks should be made before use, of the background current and also of the reading obtained with a standard long-lived source of radioactivity. Records must be kept, and any fluctuation outside statistical variation or trend in the standard value should be investigated.

Geiger counters

A Geiger counter must be operated at the mid-point of its plateau, normally about 100 V above the threshold voltage. On receipt, and prior to use if there has been an appreciable shelf-life, the plateau should be investigated. The high voltage is increased slowly until the counting starts; as the voltage is further increased the count-rate will increase sharply, and then after the threshold voltage is reached the count-rate will remain almost constant, with only a slight increase, over the plateau, which is usually about 200 V. The count-rate should be plotted against the applied voltage and the resulting curves should show the characteristics demonstrated in Fig. 3.7. The threshold voltage and length of plateau should be recorded, and the plateau slope calculated and expressed as the percentage increase in counts per 100 V increase. The background count should also be recorded, and sensitivity calibrations carried out. Weekly checks of background counts, and measurements of a long-lived reference source using a fixed geometry, should be made and recorded. If there is any trend or variation outside statistical limits (see p. 46) the plateau should be checked. If there is a significant change in threshold voltage, or plateau length or slope, the Geiger counter should be discarded.

Scintillation counters

This discussion applies to scintillation counters in general, with particular reference to those used for measurements on samples and to probe detectors. Since most currently used imaging equipment is basically scintillation-counting equipment, the general quality control is applicable. However, in view of the specialised nature of imaging equipment there are other aspects of quality control, and these will be dealt with in Chapter 7. As shown in Chapter 3, scintillation counters are usually, although not invariably, operated so that only those pulses occurring in the photopeak are selected for counting. The first step, therefore, is to find the settings corresponding to the photopeak. In the most versatile equipment there is provision for varying the settings of high voltage (HV), amplifier gain and pulse-height analyser (PHA). The first two control the amplitudes of the pulses which arrive at the input to the PHA and the last controls the range of the pulse amplitudes which are transmitted to the scaler, ratemeter, or other system, for recording.

The PHA may be calibrated by the manufacturer in volts, that is, in terms of actual pulse amplitude, or directly in keV or MeV, that is, in terms of energy of incident photon, for given settings of HV and amplifier gain. The starting point is to set the HV and amplifier gain to the recommended value and to look for a well-defined photopeak, for example of technetium-99m (photopeak

0.14 MeV). This is done by setting the channel width of the PHA to about 0.01–0.02 MeV and adjusting the threshold of the channel until the maximum count is obtained. It is wise to check that the true photopeak has been obtained by, in the case of a mono-energetic nuclide, ensuring that there are no counts above the photopeak. If necessary the HV is then adjusted to bring the ^{99m}Tc peak to a suitable value on the PHA setting. For example, if the dial or meter is calibrated directly in MeV, the HV is adjusted to bring the ^{99m}Tc peak to 0.14 MeV, whereas if the PHA control is calibrated in volts, the HV is adjusted so that as many as possible of the nuclides to be measured lie within the range of the PHA; this is of particular importance if an automatic sample-changer is to be programmed to count nuclides of different energy, since there is usually no provision for programming a change in HV. Having decided on the HV and amplifier-gain settings, the energy spectrum should be obtained for the nuclides to be measured. This is done by setting the PHA for a narrow channel width of about 2–5% of the photopeak and then taking counts for each setting of the threshold value as it is increased from its minimum value to its maximum value, or to the value at which there are no more counts. A typical energy spectrum for ^{99m}Tc has been described in Chapter 3 and is shown in Fig. 3.10. The choice of the optimum channel width for operation involves a compromise between sensitivity and resolution, and depends on the problem in hand. It is obvious that sensitivity is increased by using a wide channel, and in many sample-counting procedures sensitivity is more important than resolution. The use of a wider channel also tends to reduce variations in sensitivity. The criterion that $(C_S{}^2/C_B)$ is a maximum is useful when sensitivity is important; C_S is the source count-rate and C_B the background count-rate. For sample counting the window is usually set so that its centre is at the photopeak of the nuclide in question and its width is 20–30% of the peak energy.

Calibration factors should be obtained, via the standard ionisation chamber, for each nuclide to be used. Weekly checks of the background count, the position of the photopeak, the sensitivity using a long-lived reference source, and of within-sample variation (reproducibility of measurement on the same sample) should be carried out, and records kept. Any trends or unexpected variations should be investigated (see p. 46). In many automatic sampling units the operating conditions of the PHA are controlled by plug-in modules. With such equipment it is not possible to check the positions of the photopeaks and one must be satisfied with carrying out regular checks with long-lived standards of an energy close to that represented by the plug-in unit. The HV is usually adjusted to maintain a constant value, allowing of course for radioactive decay. A continued trend in the reference-source count must be regarded with suspicion: if it becomes necessary continuously to adjust the HV in the same direction, the system should be investigated.

After the above procedure has been carried out to establish optimum operating conditions for each nuclide, the following checks should be made.

Timing units should be checked initially for accuracy. The variation of sensitivity with sample volume should be investigated, as should the background count when an automatic sample-changer is fully loaded with samples of the nuclides to be used. The latter is of particular importance if nuclides emitting high-energy γ-radiation are to be measured. It should also be noted that when counting samples of low-energy γ-emitters, such as ^{125}I, variations in the wall thickness of the tube containing the sample may give rise to differences in absorption which could affect the accuracy of the results.

Dead-time corrections

In Chapter 3 a brief reference was made to problems which may arise in the detection of high levels of radioactivity. Such problems may arise from limitations in the detector itself, as for example in Geiger counters, or from limitations in the associated electronic equipment.

It was shown that Geiger counters have a long dead-time during which the detector is inoperable and ionising events are not detected. Because this is not constant, a paralysis time or artificial dead-time is introduced so that the counting losses can be calculated. The paralysis times used are of the order of 200–400 microseconds. Scintillation detectors are much faster, the scintillations having a half-life of about 0.2 microseconds; the limitation is usually imposed by the rate at which the pulses can be handled by the associated electronic equipment. The count-rate losses may be determined experimentally by measuring sources of increasing strength, and plotting observed count-rate against source activity (Fig. 4.1*a* and *b*). If there were no counting losses the points would lie on a straight line. The plot of true count-rate against source activity can be obtained by extrapolating the linear part of the curve at low count-rates (Fig. 4.1*a*).

The dead-time is defined as that duration of time after one detected event before the system is capable of recording the next event; during this time no second pulse gives rise to an output signal but is 'lost'. Two types of dead-time are recognised: non-paralysable and paralysable. A non-paralysable system is not influenced by these 'lost' events which occur during its recovery period, so it is inoperative for a fixed time, T, after each recorded event. In a paralysable system with a dead-time T_p, if a second event occurs during the recovery period following an event, then an additional time T_p must elapse before another event can be recorded.

The loss of counts due to the dead-time which occurs in sample counting with a non-paralysable system, may be calculated from a simple formula. If N_o counts per second are observed using counting equipment with a dead-time T, the time for which the counter is inoperative during each second will be equal to $N_o T$ seconds. Thus the proportion of counting time lost per second will be $N_o T$, and the counting time available per second will be $1 - N_o T$, that is $1/(1 - N_o T)$ of the total time.

Therefore the true count-rate N is given by

$$N = \frac{N_o}{1 - N_o T} \tag{4.1}$$

where N and N_o are expressed as counts per second and T is expressed in seconds. It follows that in Geiger counters, where

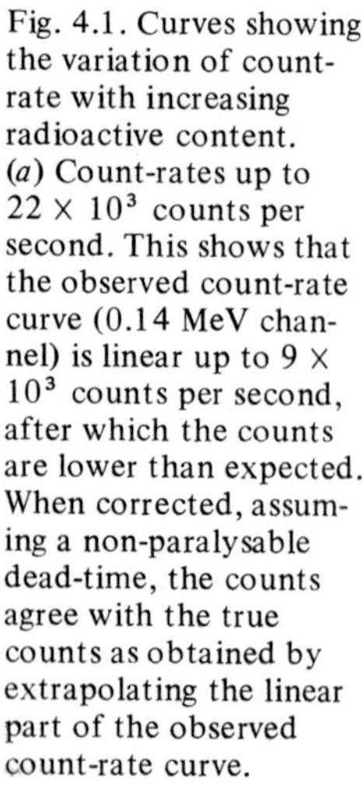

Fig. 4.1. Curves showing the variation of count-rate with increasing radioactive content. (*a*) Count-rates up to 22×10^3 counts per second. This shows that the observed count-rate curve (0.14 MeV channel) is linear up to 9×10^3 counts per second, after which the counts are lower than expected. When corrected, assuming a non-paralysable dead-time, the counts agree with the true counts as obtained by extrapolating the linear part of the observed count-rate curve.

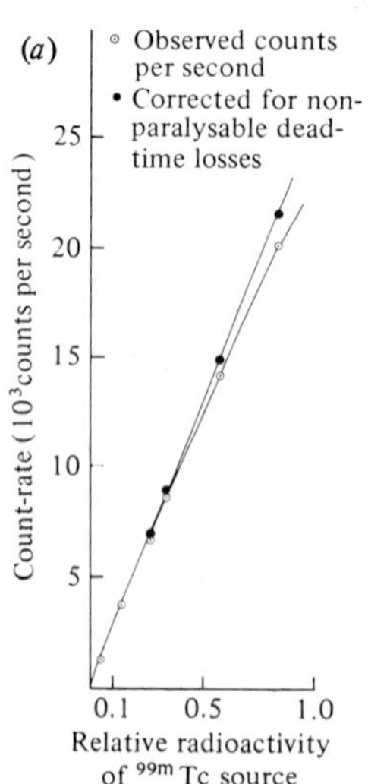

dead times are 200–400 microseconds, count losses of about 1% will occur at count-rates of 50 counts per second, whereas for scintillation counters, where overall dead-times are of the order of 1–5 microseconds, count losses only begin to become noticeable at count-rates of 5000 counts per second.

Fig. 4.1 shows the results of measurements on ^{99m}Tc sources of increasing strength, using a 7.6 cm × 7.6 cm NaI well-shaped counter. The dual-channel PHA was set so that counts were recorded simultaneously in the 0.14 MeV photopeak of ^{99m}Tc and also in a 0.28 MeV window. Both sets of observed counts were plotted against radioactivity, and it will be seen that the photopeak count-rate begins to fall off above 9×10^3 counts per second. The observed counts have been corrected for dead-time losses, assuming a non-paralysable system, using equation 4.1 and a value of 3.5 microseconds for the dead-time; the linear relationship between count-rate and activity then holds up to observed count-rates of 56×10^3 counts per second (corrected count-rates of 70.5×10^3 counts per second), when the correction is about 20%. At higher count-rates the observed photopeak count-rates fall off still more, reaching a maximum at about 110×10^3 counts per second, after which the curve turns over; when corrected for a dead-time of 3.5 microseconds the count-rates are still well below the expected values (Fig. 4.1*b*). As the photopeak

(*b*) Count-rates up to 110×10^3 counts per second. This shows that the observed counts (0.14 MeV channel) reach a maximum at 110×10^3 counts per second, after which they decrease. When corrected as in (*a*) the counts are still well below the true counts. Significant numbers of counts are observed in the 0.28 MeV channel.
(*c*) Count-rates up to 110×10^3 counts per second. This shows the same observed counts as in (*b*). The theoretical observed counts, as calculated from the extrapolated true count-rate curve assuming a paralysable dead-time, approximate to the observed counts.

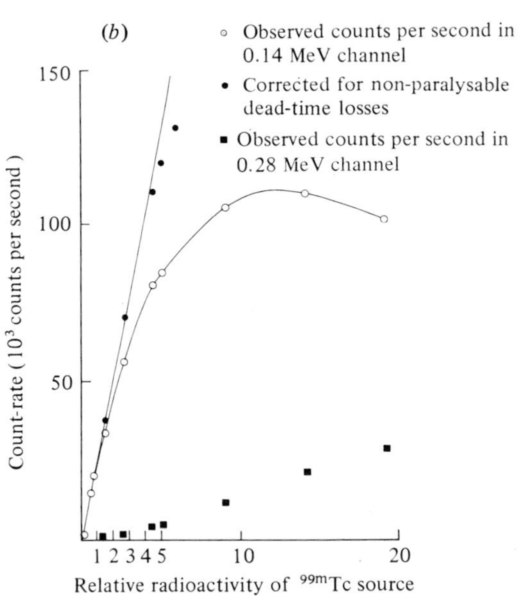

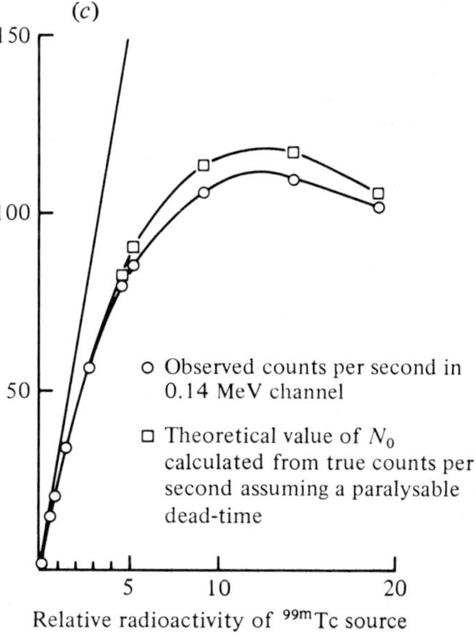

counts fall off, the number of counts in the 0.28 MeV channel starts to rise. These counts are due to pulses of twice the amplitude of the photopeak pulses, caused by the superposition of two photopeak pulses that are both detected within the resolving time of the system; it is not a simple non-paralysable system but has a paralysable component. The effect is known as the phenomenon of pile-up and occurs at very high count-rates. For a simple paralysable system the observed count-rate, N_o, of a random process such as radionuclide decay, is predicted from the Poisson distribution:

$$N_o = N\mathrm{e}^{-NT_p} \qquad (4.2)$$

where N is the true count-rate. By differentiating equation 4.2 with respect to N it can be shown that the observed count-rate passes through a maximum N_o(max) when $NT_p = 1$, and that

$$N(\mathrm{max}) = (T_p)^{-1}$$

$$\text{or } N_o(\mathrm{max}) = (\mathrm{e}T_p)^{-1} \qquad (4.3)$$

T_p can be calculated from equation 4.3, using the value of N_o(max) obtained from the experimental curve, and N calculated from equation 4.2. For both a simple paralysable system and a combined paralysable/non-paralysable system there is a maximum observed count-rate which is followed by a decrease as source strength or true count-rate increases, as shown in Fig. 4.1(*b*). At low count-rates the two-component system behaves as if only the non-paralysable component were present. There is no easy way of distinguishing between the one- and two-component systems. One difference is in the ratio N(max)/N_o(max); for a paralysable system N(max)/N_o(max) is equal to e, whereas for the two-component system N(max)/N_o(max) is greater than e.

Fig. 4.1(*c*) shows the experimental values of N_o plotted in Fig. 4.1(*b*) compared with values of N_o calculated using equations 4.2 and 4.3, and obtaining N by extrapolation of the lower part of the experimental curve. The calculated values of N_o approximate to the experimental values, showing that at high count-rates the equipment behaves as a paralysable system.

It should be noted that the number of pulses counted refers to those pulses which are within the amplitude range of the PHA window, and are therefore accepted. The γ-ray spectrum as seen by the PHA is influenced by the true count-rate, particularly at high count-rates. It was seen in Fig. 4.1(*b*) that, with a ^{99m}Tc source, pulses were counted in the 0.28 MeV window, due to superposition of two 0.14 MeV pulses; these would normally be accepted by the PHA. In the same way two pulses which would normally be rejected as being too small may overlap and be accepted. The dead-time losses of a paralysable system are therefore dependent on the PHA window, and also on the amount of scattered radiation present.

In practice, with sample counting it is not usually necessary to work with count-rates higher than about 10^4 counts per second, for which dead-time corrections are only of the order of 5%, so that the paralysable system correction is not necessary. However, in gamma cameras, where high count-rates are used in dynamic studies, these corrections become important; they will be further discussed in Chapter 7.

Decay corrections

The phenomenon of radioactive decay is discussed in Chapter 2 and, in more detail, in Chapter 10. The practical implication in sample counting is that it is important that, when relative measurements are being made, the count-rates all apply to the same moment in time; in other words, that decay corrections are applied when significant.

The count-rate N_t of a source at any time t is related to its count-rate N_0 at time t_0 by the formula

$$N_t = N_0 e^{-\lambda t} \tag{4.4}$$

where λ is the decay constant, or

$$N_t = N_0 e^{-0.693t/T_{\frac{1}{2}}} \tag{4.5}$$

where $T_{\frac{1}{2}}$ is the half-life.

The corrections may be read off decay curves (Fig. 10.4) or from tables.

Statistics

In order to be able to assess the significance of the standard checks referred to above, and of the results of radioactive counting, it is necessary to have some knowledge of statistics.

Random nature of radioactivity

If a sample of radioactive material is counted several times for the same length of time and under identical conditions, the results will not be identical. This is because radioactivity is a random process and there is no exact 'true' result. The nearest we can get to a true result is to take the mean value obtained over a long counting time. It can be shown mathematically that, for a random process in which the probability of occurrence is very small, if the count on a sample is repeated several times, and if the expected number of counts in a given time interval (that is, the average number of counts obtained over a long counting time) is equal to $\bar{N}$, then the probability of obtaining a count n in that time interval will follow a Poisson distribution.

The standard deviation, σ, for any distribution of experimental results is defined as the square root of the average of the squares of the differences of each reading from the mean, or 'root-mean-square difference'. It is a measure of experimental error.

$$\sigma = \sqrt{\left(\frac{\Sigma_1^x (\bar{N} - n)^2}{x - 1}\right)} \quad (4.6)$$

where x is the number of readings.
It can be shown mathematically that for a set of readings which follow a Poisson distribution

$$\sigma = \sqrt{\bar{N}} \quad (4.7)$$

The coefficient of variation, CV, is defined as the standard deviation divided by the mean, and is given by

$$CV = \frac{\sigma}{\bar{N}} = \frac{\sqrt{\bar{N}}}{\bar{N}} = \frac{1}{\sqrt{\bar{N}}} \quad (4.8)$$

The standard deviation of the mean, $\bar{N}$, of x readings is

$$\sigma_{\bar{N}} = \frac{\sigma}{\sqrt{(x - 1)}} \quad (4.9)$$

This equation can be used to check the consistency of the mean value obtained on weekly measurements of background and long-lived standard radioactive sources.

It can also be shown that if any series of measurements approximates to a Gaussian or normal distribution, such as is commonly encountered in natural phenomena, then 68.2% should lie within one standard deviation of the mean, and 95.4% should lie within two standard deviations of the mean. The Poisson distribution approximates to a normal distribution if a large number of readings, greater than 30, is used. It follows that if a large number of counts are taken on a radioactive sample and the average count is $\bar{N}$, then 68% should lie within $\bar{N} \pm \sqrt{\bar{N}}$, and 95% should lie within $\bar{N} \pm 2\sqrt{\bar{N}}$. The probability of a reading lying outside $\bar{N} \pm 3\sqrt{\bar{N}}$ is only 0.54%, and is therefore very remote. The expected distribution of counts is shown in Fig. 4.2. While this shows, strictly speaking, the probability that a given count will occur in a series of counts, it also indicates, approximately, the probability of the error on any single count.

The practical application of all this is that it is possible to assign a level of confidence to any count or count-rate, and also to judge the performance of counting equipment by whether or not the counts conform to the expected normal distribution. This is best shown by illustration. A series of 30 counts on a radioactive source, in equal time intervals, gave the following values:

9685	9819	10 143	9887	9805	9780
9834	9922	9961	9683	9913	9792
9938	9965	9931	9895	9825	9846
9892	9747	10 003	10 181	9773	9969
9869	9723	9711	9790	9995	9873

Mean, $\bar{N} = 9871$

Standard deviation, $\sigma = \sqrt{\bar{N}} = 99$

Number of counts lying within $\bar{N} \pm \sqrt{\bar{N}}$,
i.e. 9772 -- 9970 = 21 = 70%

Number of counts lying within $\bar{N} \pm 2\sqrt{\bar{N}}$,
i.e. 9673 − 10 071 = 28 = 93%

This is the expected distribution, and shows the equipment is functioning satisfactorily. In practice a series of 10 counts is usually considered adequate.

Fig. 4.2. Normal distribution.

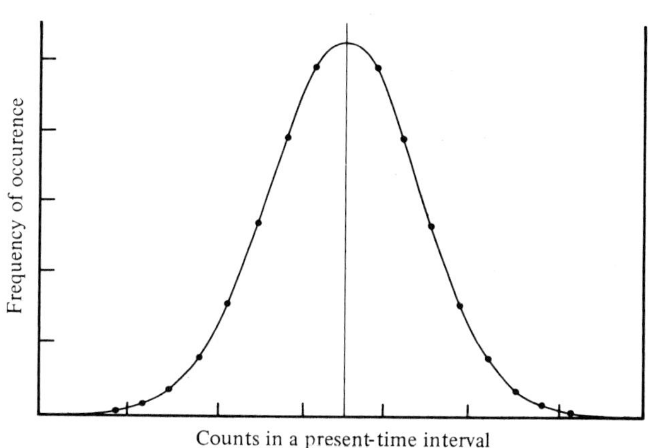

A radioactive source is counted twice for a period of 100 seconds, and counts of 10 920 and 10 760 are obtained. Is this difference of 160 acceptable? It must be said straight away that a sample of two is much too small for the application of statistical theory. But if the readings were part of a large series there should be a 95% chance that each would be within two standard deviations of the mean value, which is approximately 10 000 with a coefficient of variation of about 1%. It follows that there should be at least a 95% chance that they would be within 4% or 400 counts of each other, which they are. On another occasion two counts of 9976 and 10 554 are obtained. The difference on this occasion is 578, which is equal to nearly six standard deviations. This is suspect, and the performance and the equipment should be checked as described above.

Background-count corrections

As shown in Chapter 3, counting equipment will detect individual disintegrations; the count-rate, C_S, is proportional to radioactive content:

$$C_S = \frac{N_S}{t} \tag{4.10}$$

where N_S = number of disintegrations detected in time t

All equipment will have a background reading, C_B, due to electrical noise, cosmic radiation and other stray background radiation. If the background count-rate is significant it must be subtracted from the total count-rate:

$$C_S = C - C_B \tag{4.11}$$

where C = observed count-rate due to a sample plus background
C_B = observed background count-rate
C_S = calculated count-rate due to the sample alone

It can be shown that the standard deviation of the sum or difference of two independent values a and b is given by

$$\sigma\,(a \pm b) = \sqrt{(\sigma_a^2 + \sigma_b^2)} \tag{4.12}$$

It follows that

$$\sigma\,(C_S) = \sqrt{\{[\sigma(C)]^2 + [\sigma(C_B)]^2\}} \tag{4.13}$$

but

$$\sigma(C) = \sigma\left(\frac{N}{t}\right) \tag{4.14}$$

assuming there is no error in t,

$$\sigma(C) = \frac{\sigma(N)}{t} = \frac{\sqrt{N}}{t} = \frac{\sqrt{(Ct)}}{t} = \sqrt{\left(\frac{C}{t}\right)} \qquad (4.15)$$

therefore from equation 4.13:

$$\sigma(C_S) = \sqrt{\left(\frac{C}{t} + \frac{C_B}{t_B}\right)} \qquad (4.16)$$

The background is considered to contribute significantly to the error on C_S if its count-rate is greater than one-tenth of the sample count-rate.

If the source-plus-background and the background counts are taken over equal periods of time, then equation 4.16 reduces to

$$\sigma(N_S) = \sqrt{(N + N_B)} \qquad (4.17)$$

The limit of sensitivity of any piece of sample-counting equipment is determined by the background. Veall (1971) has shown that if the sensitivity is defined as the lowest sample activity which can be detected with 99% confidence in a single measurement, then it is that activity which gives a count-rate equal to one-tenth of the background count.

Relative count-rates

In most measurements of radioactivity one is concerned with relative count-rates, e.g. expressing the radioactivity in an unknown sample relative to that in an accurately prepared standard, or observing the changes in radioactivity in samples taken over a period of time. The coefficient of variation, CV (the standard deviation divided by the mean) of a ratio (or a product) of two variables a and b is given by

$$CV\left(\frac{a}{b}\right) = CV(ab) = \sqrt{[CV(a)]^2 + [CV(b)]^2} \qquad (4.18)$$

This equation is similar to equation 4.12 which calculates the standard deviation on the difference between two variables, except that the coefficient of variation is used throughout instead of the standard deviation.

Optimisation of counting time

In order to use equipment to the best advantage, counting times need to be reduced to the minimum that is necessary to achieve the required accuracy. It is generally not optimal from this point of view to count samples (including background) and background for the same length of time. It can be shown that the optimum distribution of time between sample and background counting times is in direct ratio to the square roots of the count-rates, C, as shown in the following equation:

$$\frac{t}{t_B} = \frac{\sqrt{C}}{\sqrt{C_B}} \tag{4.19}$$

Similarly it can be shown that the optimum distribution of counting times when the ratio of the activities of two samples is required, is given by

$$\frac{t_1}{t_2} = \frac{\sqrt{C_2}}{\sqrt{C_1}} \tag{4.20}$$

Although of importance when using manual counters, these considerations may not be very relevant to automatic sample-changers, unless there is a large number of small batches of samples, with each batch requiring a background, and the system is readily programmable to count for different times. With such systems there is usually an alternative arrangement whereby all samples can be counted until a pre-set number of counts is obtained, e.g. up to 10 000 counts to give a 1% coefficient of variation. There is usually also a pre-set limit to the counting time, e.g. 100 or 400 seconds, so that if the count-rate is very low, say 10 counts per second, the count will be terminated after 400 seconds when 4000 counts are collected, giving a 2% coefficient of variation, instead of continuing to 1000 seconds.

This reasoning of optimisation has been further pursued by R.P. Ekins (personal communication), who has considered the logistics of counting times as applied in particular to single large batches of samples in radioimmunoassay work. He has worked out a system whereby an acceptable standard deviation is agreed, for any particular hormone assay, and also for any particular level of that hormone. For instance, levels which are well above or well below normal require less accuracy than those which are borderline. The counting times are optimised to obtain these accepted levels of confidence. The argument in the preceding paragraph applies purely to the optimisation of counting times in relation to the statistical counting errors caused by the random nature of radioactivity. The theory of errors states that if the individual percentage probable errors in an experiment are $E_1, E_2, E_3, \ldots, E_n$, then the overall percentage probable error is given by

$E = \sqrt{(E_1^2 + E_2^2 + E_3^2 + \ldots E_n^2)}$, provided that the individual measurements are independent of each other. Ekins has considered the statistical errors in relation to the other experimental errors, e.g. pipetting errors, and has also looked at the overall error on each sample in the context of the clinical significance of the final result. More specifically, by the use of microprocessors, he feeds the estimated experimental error, excluding statistical errors, into the counting system and uses an equation to calculate the additional statistical error which would increase the overall error on any result by a definite amount (e.g. 50%) to the accepted minimum acceptable error for that result. The count-rate obtained over the first few seconds is used to calculate the result, and the minimum acceptable error for that result is then sought; the allowable statistical error is then calculated and the counting time can be set accordingly. Ekins claims that using these techniques the counting times can be reduced significantly from those required when working to fixed statistical errors.

Summary of corrections to be applied

(1) Dead-time correction: this applies to the total observed count-rate.
(2) Background correction.
(3) Decay correction: this applies to the source count-rate.

The above should be applied if they are greater than the standard deviation of the result.

References

Veall, N. (1971). Statistical factors affecting radioactivity measurements. In *Radioisotopes in Medical Diagnosis*, ed. E.H. Belcher & H. Vetter, pp. 70–1. London: Butterworth.

5. Radiopharmaceuticals

Definition

A radiopharmaceutical is any radioactive product which is administered to a human being for medicinal purposes, usually investigational, in which the radioactivity is an essential part of the product.

Development

There has been a tremendous and rapid development in this field over the past two decades. Prior to 1960 the use of radiopharmaceuticals was restricted almost entirely to nuclides produced by neutron irradiation, for example iodine-131 for thyroid investigations, chromium-51 for red cell labelling and iron-59 for iron turnover studies. In 1953 the first medical cyclotron was built at Hammersmith Hospital and in 1956 the 23 MeV cyclotron at Oak Ridge National Laboratory was used to produce short-lived radionuclides for clinical work.

The commercial development of generator systems to produce short-lived radionuclides from long-lived parent nuclides began in 1954, and the technetium-99m generator in particular has had a dramatic impact on imaging techniques. In 1965 a symposium on radioactive pharmaceuticals was held at Oak Ridge, Tennessee (USAEC, 1966) which brought together people of diverse backgrounds and interests: physicists, biochemists, pharmacologists, nuclear-medicine clinicians, and representatives from the fields of radionuclide production, from the radiopharmaceutical industry and from government regulatory agencies. Radiopharmacy emerged as a discipline. The International Atomic Energy Agency convened a panel of experts in May 1970, and jointly with the World Health Organisation arranged a symposium in March 1975. The proceedings of both these meetings are published (IAEA, 1971, 1975) and provide good guidelines on fundamental principles. Meanwhile, in the UK the preparation of radiopharmaceuticals developed on a rather *ad hoc* basis. In 1968 the Medicines Act was passed in the UK to introduce a system of controls over the manufacture and distribution of medicinal products, and the Act caused the question of radiopharmaceuticals to be considered in a new light. A joint meeting between the Pharmaceutical Society and the Hospital Physicists' Association was called in 1970, to discuss the preparation of radiopharmaceuticals. Two sets of guidelines have been published (BIR, 1975; HPA, 1977), both of which give much valuable information.

Requirements for a good radiopharmaceutical

Obviously the ideal requirements for the radiopharmaceutical will vary to a certain extent with the type of study, but there are common factors. Firstly, the radiation dose to the patient must be kept as low as possible. Secondly, if external measurements are to be made, the radiation emitted must be sufficiently energetic to penetrate to the surface of the body and of the correct energy to give a good response in the detecting equipment. Thirdly, the radiopharmaceutical must have the correct physiological properties. Finally, it must be readily obtainable and reasonably cheap.

The first two factors above are determined mainly by the physical properties of the radionuclide, that is the type and energy of radiation emitted and the half-life of the radionuclide, but since the operative half-life for dosage calculation is the effective half-life, the biological half-life is also important. As will be seen in Chapter 11 particulate radiation gives a much greater dose than electromagnetic radiation, and has a very short range. It is evident, therefore, that this is unwanted radiation when external detection is required; it contributes to a high dose but serves no useful purpose. The ideal nuclide will emit γ-radiation of appropriate energy but no particulate radiation; that is, it will decay by isomeric transition, or electron capture. Most detectors are basically scintillation counters with NaI crystals, and require lead collimation. The optimum energy for such detectors is 0.12–0.16 MeV for gamma cameras and 0.14–0.35 MeV for other scintillation detectors.

The optimum half-life varies with the investigation; since it is obvious that sufficient radioactivity must persist until measurements are completed, it is the shortest half-life compatible with this requirement. If, however, the biological half-life is short, the radiation dose is governed by this, and the physical half-life is unimportant. Some examples may help to clarify the above.

Consider the radiopharmaceuticals which have been used in bone investigations: strontium-85, strontium-87m, calcium-47, fluorine-18, and technetium-99m labelled phosphate compounds. The physical properties of these nuclides, and the radiation to bone received per microcurie administered intravenously, are shown in Table 5.1.

Obviously for metabolic studies it is preferable to use isotopes of elements which are bone constituents. ^{45}Ca, being a pure β-emitter, cannot be detected externally but has been used for studies of bone metabolism in animals by doing autoradiography on bone samples. Short-term and long-term metabolic studies using external counting have been carried out using ^{47}Ca and ^{85}Sr respectively; both of these give high radiation doses, which means that the amount administered to humans must be limited, and most investigators have used 0.5–1 μCi of ^{85}Sr per kilogram of body weight, that is 35–70 μCi for the average patient. For imaging, as regards metabolism it is only important that the radioactive material be taken up by, or deposited in, bone; fluorine is said to be taken up in bone by ionic exchange because of its similarity to the hydroxyl ion, and the phosphate compounds have been shown to be deposited in bone. An additional requirement for imaging of bone is a short-lived γ-emitting nuclide; the imaging is normally carried out 2 to 4 hours after the administration, as soon as the radiopharmaceutical is cleared from the blood and taken up by bone. Those used include ^{87m}Sr, ^{18}F, and ^{99m}Tc phosphate compounds. As seen from the table these give radiation doses of the order of 100 times less than ^{47}Ca and ^{85}Sr; much larger quantities can therefore be given, and usual amounts are 2 mCi of ^{87m}Sr, 2 mCi of ^{18}F and 15 mCi of ^{99m}Tc, resulting in much better counting statistics.

Preparation of radiopharmaceuticals

It is not proposed to give details of any preparations, partly because these are always changing and new materials are continually being developed. Each preparation must have a Master Control Document, of which all staff involved in the preparations should be given a copy; it should contain detailed instructions of preparation and quality control. Examples of Master Control Docu-

Table 5.1 *Physical properties of radionuclides used in bone investigations*

	^{45}Ca	^{47}Ca	^{85}Sr	^{87m}Sr	^{18}F	^{99m}Tc
Physical half-life	163 days	4.5 days	65 days	2.8 hours	1.8 hours	6 hours
Primary mode of decay and energy (MeV)	β^- 0.257	β^- 0.688 (82%) 1.985 (18%)	Electron capture	Electron capture	β^+ 0.250	Isomeric transition
Photon energy (MeV)	None	0.489 (6.8%) 0.808 (6.8%) 1.297 (75%)	0.514	0.388	0.511	0.14
Bone radiation dose						
rad mCi^{-1} (approx.)	370	55	120	0.3	0.5	0.2
Gy GBq^{-1} (approx.)	100	15	32	0.081	0.13	0.054

ments are given in the appendix to this chapter (p. 72).

The facilities required for different types of preparation are discussed in the two sets of guidelines mentioned earlier (BIR, 1975; HPA, 1977), and the reader is referred to these. However, a few general points may be made.

The preparation area must provide an environment where the risk of radiation hazard to the staff and the risk of microbial and particulate contamination of the products intended for injection into patients are acceptably low. The facilities required will obviously vary with the size of the department and the scope of the work; in general a clean room containing an aseptic area will be the minimum requirement. A clean room is so designed to prevent accumulation of dust and render cleaning easy, and includes an entry lobby with changing facilities for staff. It should have a filtered air intake to remove at least 99% of particles down to 5 μm in diameter, and ventilation to produce eight room air changes per hour and to maintain a positive pressure of 12–37 pascals. The aseptic area may be a separate room within the clean room, but usually a special type of laminar, or unidirectional, airflow cabinet will suffice. The essential feature of the cabinet is the creation of a column of filtered air moving through the cabinet with a uniform velocity of about 0.5 m per second, thus providing a virtually particle-free environment. In order to provide radiological protection for the operator from airborne material, particularly when volatile substances are being used, air must also be drawn *inwards* through the working aperture. Because this is not filtered air it must be directed within the cabinet so that it does not pass over the preparation. Adequate lead or lead glass shielding must be provided where necessary to keep the radiation exposure within acceptable levels.

Specification of purity and quality control

There are four aspects of purity which need to be considered. These are chemical, radiochemical, radionuclide and pharmaceutical, and they will be considered separately.

Chemical purity and specific activity

Chemical purity is defined as the fraction of the total mass that is present in the stated chemical form. Chemical impurities do not usually present a problem. However, since radiopharmaceuticals often employ the rarer elements, it is important that toxicity checks are carried out before a new product is used clinically. It should be borne in mind that the amount of the radioactive substance present is very small (for example 10 mCi of ^{99m}Tc, if carrier-free, weighs only 2×10^{-9} g), and therefore all the precautions which relate to the handling of very dilute solutions are applicable. Any minute trace of an impurity is liable to affect labelling efficiency and reproducibility, but it is difficult to detect such impurities and therefore all reasonable steps should be taken to ensure that the chemical purity is of an acceptable standard. Some of the commercially available longer-lived radiopharmaceuticals contain bacteriostats; this is clearly stated on the label.

The specific activity of the product is defined as the fraction of the total active ingredient in radioactive form, and is expressed as mCi mg^{-1} (MBq mg^{-1}). Specific activity is often important in tracer studies, since administration of a large quantity of the compound may distort the metabolic process under investigation.

Radiochemical purity

This is usually defined as the percentage of the stated radioactivity which is in the stated chemical form. Radiochemical purity is important in quantitative studies and in imaging, because it is assumed that all the radioactivity administered is in the correct chemical form and will behave accordingly. If this is not so, and a significant part of the radioactivity is in a different chemical form, it will behave differently and results may be invalidated. Moreover a different distribution and clearance rate may give rise to an unnecessary radiation dose. For example, in renographic studies, if a significant proportion of ^{131}I were in the form of free iodide instead of being incorporated into hippuran, the result would be affected because the clearance from the blood is much slower for free iodide than for hippuran. Moreover, the free iodide would be selectively taken up by the thyroid, giving an unsuspected radiation dose, unless the thyroid was blocked by prior administration of potassium iodide. Another example is that of lung imaging. For this investigation macroaggregates or microspheres of human serum albumin (HSA) of diameter 15–20 μm are labelled with ^{99m}Tc, injected intravenously, and become trapped in the lung capillaries. If the particles are too small they will not be trapped in the lung but will be removed by the reticulo-endothelial system, and the liver will then be imaged instead of the lung. If free ^{99m}Tc is present it will be trapped by the thyroid gland and a thyroid image will result; there will, moreover, be a high blood background present.

Radionuclidic purity

This is defined as the percentage of the total radioactivity which is present as the stated radionuclide. The impurity may be isotopic with the stated radionuclide; for example ^{123}I when produced by bombardment of antimony with 25 MeV α-particles is significantly contaminated with ^{124}I. Alternatively, the impurity may be a different element from the stated radionuclide; for example ^{99m}Tc obtained from a generator may be contaminated with ^{99}Mo if break-through has occurred. If radionuclide impurities are present in commercially available materials, this will be clearly stated. With generators it is essential to check the eluates for contamination, and this will be dealt with in more detail in the section on generators (p. 66).

It should be noted that radionuclidic purity is not constant. If the half-life of the contaminant is greater than the half-life of the stated nuclide, the degree of contamination increases with time, and this is very important in relation to the radiation dose to the patient. For example, the half-life of ^{123}I is 13 hours while that of ^{124}I is 4.2 days, so that after 26 hours the ^{123}I is reduced to 25% of its original value whereas the ^{124}I is only reduced to 85%. An initial ^{124}I contamination of 5% will therefore be increased to 14% after one day's storage. The presence of long-lived contaminants increases the radiation dose unnecessarily, and if they cannot be eliminated their contribution to the patient-dose must be taken into account.

Pharmaceutical purity

Most radiopharmaceuticals are administered by intravenous injection and must therefore comply with the normal requirements for injections, i.e. the solution must be sterile, free from pyrogens and foreign particulate matter, and of acceptable pH.

Commercially produced radiopharmaceuticals

There are many firms which produce radiopharmaceuticals, but in the UK The Radiochemical Centre, Amersham, has the monopoly. In the UK all manufacturers or manufacturers' agents are now required, in order to conform with the Medicines Act, to hold a product licence for every product on the market; the licensing authority is the Department of Health and Social Security. It can be assumed that radiopharmaceuticals purchased from a manufacturer will have a product licence and will conform to the accepted standards for quality, although this should be checked for new materials.

Radiopharmaceuticals with a long half-life, that is greater than 12 hours, present no problem. The guaranteed radiochemical and radionuclidic purity of the product will be stated in the catalogue or sales literature, and any tests of these done by the user will be corroborative only. The radioactivity on the reference date, the volume, the specific activity (unless the product is sold as carrier-free) and an expiry date (if relevant) will be stated on each individual container of radioactive material. The radioactivity of each source should be checked on receipt. If the solution is in a multi-dose vial, it must either be dispensed out into single-dose, sterile, pyrogen-free vials, under sterile conditions, or it must be re-autoclaved after each entry. The choice between these two methods will be determined by whether or not the solution is stable under autoclave conditions. Each individual dose must be measured before administration to check its radioactivity, and must be clearly labelled. It is important to know whether any special storage conditions are necessary; some solutions, e.g. labelled human serum albumin and labelled cyanocobalamin, must be stored in a refrigerator at 5 °C, and others are sensitive to light. If not stored under the specified conditions there may be problems as a result of breakdown of the product or bacterial growth. Substances which are known to be unstable should be checked for radiochemical purity before use.

Generators

The term generator is applied to a system which provides a regular supply of a short-lived nuclide. A long-lived nuclide which is the parent of a decay series, is absorbed on to an alumina or resin column. It decays to the required short-lived nuclide and at equilibrium, which is reached at about four half-lives of the daughter, the activity of the daughter-product is equal to the activity of the parent. The daughter-product can be eluted off by running the appropriate solvent through the alumina column, leaving the parent nuclide behind. The activity of the daughter-product is then built up again on the column as the parent decays; the activity available for elution will depend on the time elapsed since the previous elution. Thus a regular supply of the short-lived nuclide is available until the parent nuclide decays below the required level. A drawing and a photograph of a typical technetium generator are shown in Fig. 5.1.

The decay of the parent nuclide and the growth of the daughter can be expressed mathematically and the scheme for a ^{99m}Tc

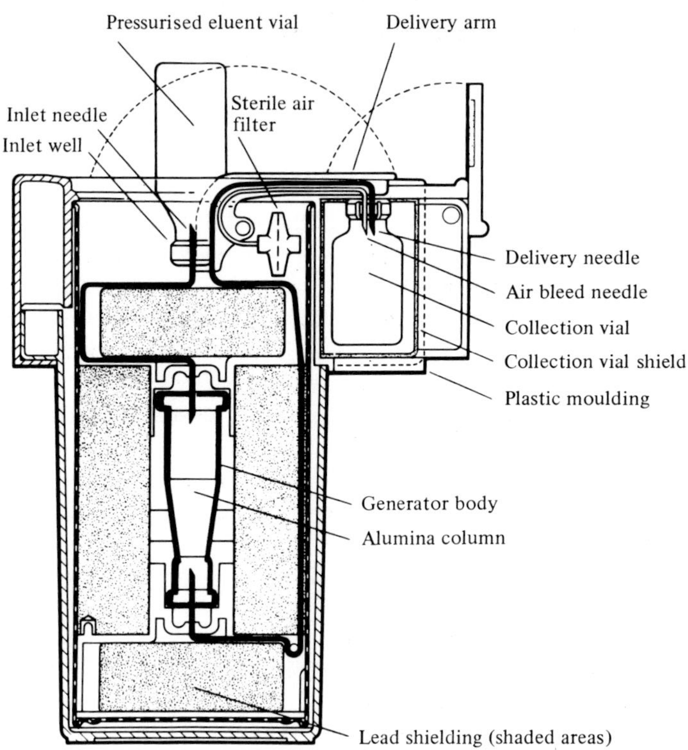

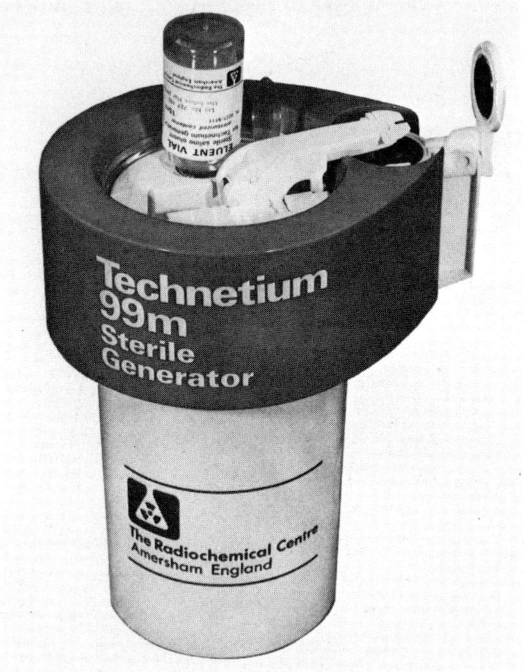

Fig. 5.1. Drawing and photograph of a ^{99m}Tc generator. (Kindly provided by The Radiochemical Centre.)

generator is shown in Fig. 5.2. The parent nuclide molybdenum-99 (A), decays with a disintegration constant λ_A to form, in 90% of disintegrations, a daughter-product technetium-99m (B) which in turn decays, with a disintegration constant λ_B, to technetium-99. In the other 10% of disintegrations ^{99}Mo decays directly to ^{99}Tc. We shall consider the 90% disintegration path.

The decay of ^{99}Mo may be expressed as

$$\frac{dN_A}{dt} = -\lambda_A N_A \tag{5.1}$$

or

$$N_A = N_0 e^{-\lambda_A t} \tag{5.2}$$

The rate of growth of ^{99m}Tc is equal to 90% of the rate of decay of ^{99}Mo less its own rate of decay. Therefore

$$\frac{dN_B}{dt} = 0.9\lambda_A N_A - \lambda_B N_B \tag{5.3}$$

$$= 0.9\lambda_A N_0 e^{-\lambda_A t} - \lambda_B N_B \tag{5.4}$$

The solution of this differential equation is

$$\frac{N_B}{N_0} = \frac{0.9\lambda_A}{\lambda_B - \lambda_A}(e^{-\lambda_A t} - e^{-\lambda_B t}) \tag{5.5}$$

and therefore

$$\frac{A_B}{A_0} = \frac{0.9\lambda_B}{\lambda_B - \lambda_A}(e^{-\lambda_A t} - e^{-\lambda_B t}) \tag{5.6}$$

where

$$A = \text{radioactivity} = \frac{dN}{dt} = \lambda N.$$

Equation 5.6 expresses the activity of the daughter product B, at any time t, as a fraction of the activity of the parent A at t_0, the time immediately after elution when there is no activity due to *B*. From equation 5.2

$$A_A = A_0 e^{-\lambda_A t} \tag{5.7}$$

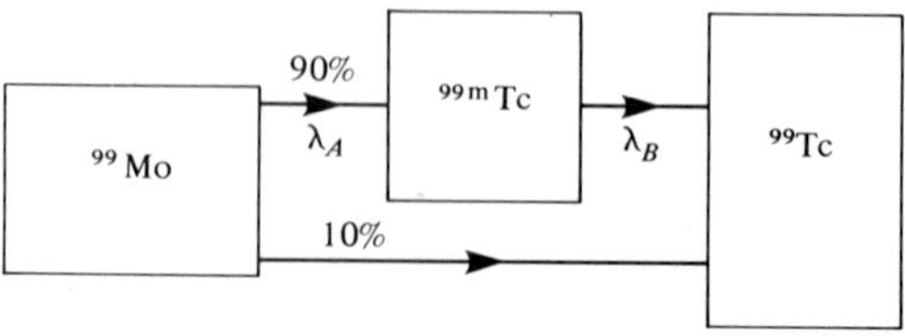

Fig. 5.2. Decay scheme for ^{99m}Tc generator.

which expresses the activity of the parent product A at any time t. Using equations 5.6 and 5.7, and the decay constant λ_A equal to 0.0103 per hour for ^{99}Mo ($T_{\frac{1}{2}} = 67$ hours), and λ_B equal to 0.1155 per hour for ^{99m}Tc ($T_{\frac{1}{2}} = 6$ hours), it is possible to calculate the activity of the ^{99}Mo in the generator, at any time after the reference time, and the percentage of the equilibrium ^{99m}Tc activity at any time interval after elution.

Fig. 5.3(*a*) shows the decay curve for ^{99}Mo plotted on a log-linear scale. It will be seen that it has fallen to about one-fifth of its original value after 7 days, so that 1 week constitutes its useful life. Fig. 5.3(*b*) shows the decay curve of ^{99}Mo and the growth curve of ^{99m}Tc calculated from equations 5.7 and 5.6 respectively. These may be used to calculate the available ^{99m}Tc in a given situation; for example, a generator delivered on a Monday, with nominal activity 100 mCi, has been eluted at 08.30 hours on a Thursday; more ^{99m}Tc is urgently required at 12.00 hours. What activity is available immediately, and what would be gained by waiting another 2 hours? Curve (*a*) shows that on Thursday, after 3 days, the ^{99}Mo activity would be 47%, that is 47 mCi. Curve (*b*) shows that 3½ hours after elution only 30%, that is 14.2 mCi, would be available, but that by waiting another 2 hours 41% (i.e. 19 mCi) would be available. A calculator is provided with the Radiochemical Centre generator which enables the value of A_B multiplied by A_A to be read off directly (Fig. 5.4).

Many generators are now available and they are listed in Table 5.2. The two most widely used are the technetium-99m and the

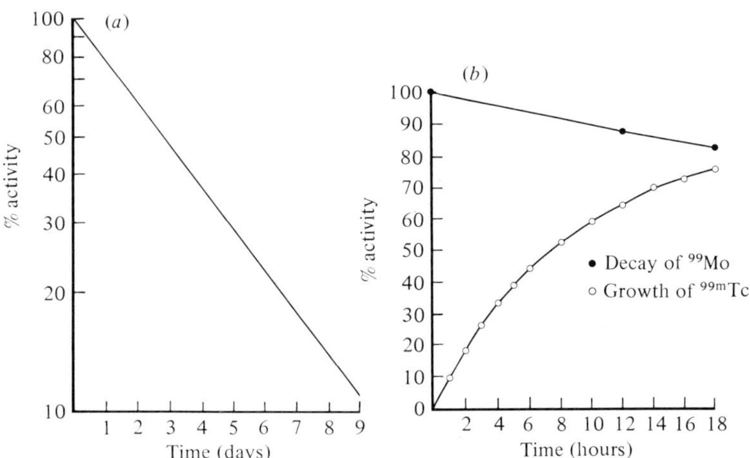

Fig. 5.3. (*a*) Decay curve for ^{99}Mo plotted on log-linear scale. (*b*) Decay curve for ^{99}Mo plotted on linear scale and growth curve of ^{99m}Tc.

TO CALCULATE 99mTc
ON THE GENERATOR COLUMN
1 Set arrow A to elution time on the outer disc
2 Set arrow B to time since previous elution on the middle disc
3 Set cursor line to generator size on the inner disc
4 Read off the 99mTc activity from the outer scale
Note: the activity of technetium-99m that can be obtained from the generator will depend on the elution efficiency
To calculate the decay of 99mTc and 99Mo use the cursor scales together with the outer mCi scale
Technetium-99m
Sterile Generator Activity Calculator
The Radiochemical Centre
Amersham
England
Generator size at reference (mCi)
Time since previous elution (hours)
Time of elution from reference date
Time of day (hours GMT)
Days from reference
Reference date
mCi
99mTc (Hours)
99Mo (Hours)

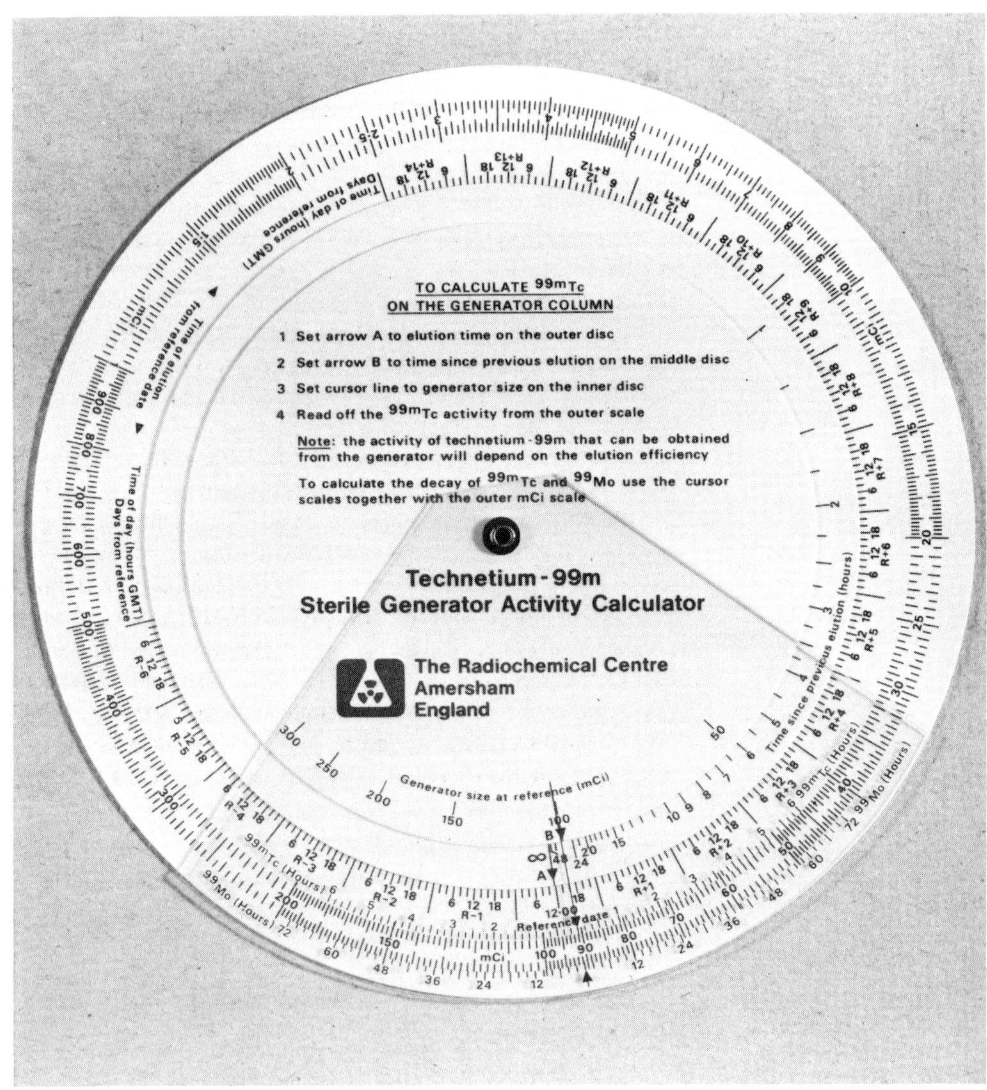

Fig. 5.4. Calculator for use with ^{99m}Tc generator.

indium-113m generators; both of these nuclides may be used in appropriate chemical forms to image most of the important organs.

The development of generators has had a tremendous impact on imaging techniques, because it has made practicable the use of short-lived nuclides. It is now possible to administer millicurie amounts of radiopharmaceuticals, rather than microcurie amounts as with the long-lived nuclides; this of course gives much better statistics. However, there are problems connected with the preparation of radiopharmaceuticals from generator products which do not arise with the longer-lived nuclides, since the latter are subjected to quality control by the manufacturer before dispatch. Although the manufacturer of the generator can carry out quality control checks on a batch of generators before dispatch, and can claim that if the generator is handled correctly the eluate will conform to the specified standards of radiochemical, radionuclidic and pharmaceutical quality, the final responsibility rests with the consumer. It is therefore incumbent on the person responsible – the physicist, pharmacist or clinician – to establish a rigid procedure of preparation, and to set out a series of quality control checks which will ensure that a high standard is maintained. It must be appreciated that some of the results of the

Table 5.2 *Radionuclide generators now available*

Daughter or product radionuclide	Half-life	Primary mode of decay[a]	Photon energy (MeV)	Parent nuclide and half-life	Use
^{99m}Tc	6 hours	IT	0.14	^{99}Mo 2.7 days	Multiple (see text)
^{113m}In	1.67 hours	IT	0.392	^{113}Sn 118 days	Multiple
^{87}Sr	2.8 hours	IT	0.388	^{87}Y 3.33 days	Bone imaging
^{68}Ga	1.13 hours	EC	0.511 (annihilation)	^{68}Ge 287 days	Bone, brain, kidney and liver imaging
^{81m}Kr	13 seconds	IT	0.191	^{81}Rb 4.7 hours	Lung-ventilation perfusion studies
^{137m}Ba	2.5 minutes	IT	0.661	^{137}Cs 30 years	Cardiac output measurement circulation studies
^{103m}Rh	57 minutes	IT	0.0397	^{103}Pd 17 days	
^{132}I	2.3 hours	β^-	0.523 0.630 and others	^{132}Te 3.2 days	Thyroid function studies
^{191m}Ir	4.9 seconds	IT	0.129	^{191}Os 15.3 days	Cardiac studies

[a]EC, electron capture; IT, isomeric transition. (See Glossary for details.)

quality control, particularly for pharmaceutical quality, will only be available retrospectively, that is after the material has been administered to the patient. Meticulous adherence to the procedure laid down is essential with regard to the details of the preparation, to the radiation protection rules, and to quality control checks.

Technetium-99m generator and compounds

Technetium-99m has been widely accepted as the radionuclide of choice for many investigations. This is because it has ideal physical properties for imaging, particularly with gamma cameras. Its decay is by isomeric transition, so there is no nuclear particulate radiation but only an almost mono-energetic γ-radiation of 0.14 MeV, although it must be appreciated that there are some internal conversion electrons. These radiation characteristics, combined with its short half-life of 6 hours, result in a low radiation dose to the patient. Moreover the photon energy of 0.14 MeV gives a high detection efficiency with the thin crystal of a gamma camera. As seen in Table 3.2 the efficiency is 100% for γ-radiation of 0.14 MeV, with crystals of 1.27 cm thickness or greater. Collimation is readily achieved since the half-value-layer (HVL) in lead is only 0.25 mm, and 1 mm and 2 mm of lead reduce the intensity to 6.8 and 0.48% respectively. The preparation of ^{99m}Tc from the ^{99}Mo generator ensures that it is readily available.

Technetium generators were first used in 1964. The ^{99}Mo used was produced by neutron irradiation of ^{98}Mo in a reactor, and because of the non-availability of very high flux reactors or supplies of enriched target material, the product, $(n, \gamma)^{99}$Mo, was generally of low specific activity. While this is adequate and widely used for generators in small centres, the development, in many countries, of large radiopharmaceutical laboratories to supply several smaller centres, and the need for small-volume injections in dynamic techniques, have led to a demand for high-activity generators and high eluate concentrations. The disadvantage of low specific activity $(n, \gamma)^{99}$Mo is that, because the amount of material that can be adsorbed on to an alumina bed is limited, in order to get a high-activity generator it is necessary to use a large bed size, with consequent problems of shielding, and a low concentration eluate. $(n, f)^{99}$Mo may be obtained carrier-free as a fission product, and this is used in the so-called fission ^{99m}Tc generators; these may carry ^{99}Mo activities of several curies yielding high concentration eluates, and are used in large central radiopharmacies. Alternatively eluates of suitable quality may be obtained from low-flux-irradiated natural molybdenum trioxide by sublimation or solvent extraction of the ^{99m}Tc from ^{99}Mo.

Radiation protection. Technetium generators using (n, γ)^{99m}Tc are available with activities ranging from 25 mCi to 400 mCi on the reference day and those using (n, f)^{99m}Tc with up to 2 Ci; most manufacturers deliver 2 or 3 days before the reference day, so the generator may contain up to twice its nominal value on receipt. Generators with activities up to 800 mCi (n, γ)^{99}Mo in equilibrium with 800 mCi ^{99m}Tc, or 4 Ci (n, f)^{99}Mo in equilibrium with 4 Ci ^{99m}Tc may therefore be encountered. All modern generators are housed in lead shielding, as shown in Fig. 5.1 where the thickness of lead is 30 mm, which reduces the 0.74 and 0.78 MeV radiation of ^{99}Mo to 4% of the unscreened value. Some manufacturers, for example Duphar Ltd, provide additional lead screening for high-activity generators. The radiation exposure at the surface of the generator, and also at working distance, should be measured by the radiation safety officer of the department, and should be displayed so that all staff are informed; at the working distance it should be less than the maximum permissible rate, that is 3 mR per hour for a 35 hour week. Typical values are: at 50 cm from a 200 mCi RCC generator, about 3 mR per hour; and at 50 cm from a 600 mCi Duphar generator, with no extra shielding or in a second lead enclosure, 10 mR per hour and less than 0.5 mR per hour respectively. The 0.14 MeV γ-radiation of ^{99m}Tc is readily shielded, giving acceptable levels, as shown in Table 11.5.

Pharmaceutical quality. Generators are guaranteed sterile and free from pyrogens when despatched, but strict attention must be paid to aseptic techniques to ensure that they remain sterile; even so there is a difference of opinion as to whether they can be considered to be sterile throughout their lives, if full aseptic conditions do not prevail. It has been suggested that generators should be housed in laminar flow cabinets, but it is generally considered that a clean room is adequate. The procedure for maintenance of aseptic working conditions should be clearly set out in the master document, and this procedure must be strictly adhered to.

Radioactive content of eluate. The generator is usually eluted first thing in the morning, and the manufacturer's instructions must be followed exactly. The expected activity will be known, and if the measured activity does not agree with this an explanation must be sought, if necessary from the manufacturer.

Radionuclide purity. There is usually ^{99}Mo in the eluate, and a check for this ^{99}Mo break-through must be made daily before using the eluate to prepare patient-doses, to ensure that the ^{99m}Tc is not contaminated with ^{99}Mo. This is most easily done by measuring the radioactivity with and without a 4 mm lead filter. The ^{99m}Tc radiation being of lower energy (0.14 MeV) it will be almost completely absorbed by the lead filter, whereas the higher-energy ^{99}Mo radiation (0.37–0.78 MeV) will only be reduced to about 30%. The activity measured with the lead filter is therefore the activity due to ^{99}Mo. For example, the radiation from a 200 mCi ^{99m}Tc eluate will be reduced to 0.001%, that is to the equivalent of 2 μCi, whereas that from a 0.05% molybdenum contamination, 100 μCi, would only be reduced to the equivalent of 30 μCi, and the latter would be measured with the filter in position. The Radiochemical Centre claims at least 99.9% radionuclidic purity, and less than 0.1% of ^{99}Mo contamination of the eluate up to 8 hours after elution. If the ^{99}Mo content exceeds 0.05% at the time of elution, the eluate should not be used, and the manufacturers consulted.

Chemical purity. The eluate should be checked for the presence of alumina, which may break through from the alumina bed. The test is a simple colorimetric test using Mordant Blue III, which should be carried out before the generator is put into use.

Compounds. The eluate contains ^{99m}Tc in the form of pertechnetate, $^{99m}TcO_4$, and this is used for some applications, such as thyroid and brain imaging. For other investigations it is necessary to obtain the ^{99m}Tc in a chemical form which has the right physiological behaviour. Those forms commonly used are shown in Table 5.3. For most of these preparations 'kits' are commercially available, and the preparation merely involves adding one solution to another under aseptic conditions. Some examples of preparation are given in the master documents in the appendix at the end of the chapter (p. 72).

Records

Records must be kept of all radionuclides which come into the department, and of all radioactive waste disposal (see appendix to Chapter 11, p. 215). All long-lived nuclides should be assayed for radioactivity on receipt, and a record kept of subsequent use. A book should be kept for each generator to record the activity obtained at each elution, and the compounds and individual doses prepared with each elution. All radioactive solutions, including patient-doses, must be clearly labelled at the time of preparation. Good pharmaceutical practice demands that it must be possible to trace the source of every component in every individual dose, and to this end batch numbers of all components must be recorded. Each patient-dose must be accompanied by a form which states the patient's name, the test requested, the radionuclide and chemical form, the date, the activity at a specified time, and the volume; the form must be initialled by the person who prepared it. Before the dose is given the information on this form must be checked against that on the investigation request form, to which it is then attached, and the patient identified by both surname and Christian name. Finally the form is signed by the person giving the injection or oral dose. A central card index record should be kept, with a card for each patient recording all administrations of radioactive doses. There should also be a record in the patient's notes.

Cyclotron-produced nuclides

Another source of short-lived radionuclides is the cyclotron. There are now about 60 commercial cyclotrons in the world.

Table 5.3 *^{99m}Tc labelled compounds and other substances in general use*

Substance	Use
Antimony sulphide colloid Sulphur colloid Tin colloid	Liver imaging
Macroaggregates of human serum albumin (MAA) Microspheres of human serum albumin	Lung imaging
Pyrophosphate (Pyro P), Polyphosphate (Poly P) Ethylenehydroxydiphosphonate (EHDP) Methylenediphosphonate (MDP), imidodiphosphate (IDP)	Bone imaging
Dimercocaptosuccinate (DMSA)	Kidney imaging
Diethylenetriaminepentaacetate (tin) [DTPA (Sn)]	Renography
Red cells	Measurement of red cell volume
Sphered red cells	Spleen imaging

Apart from the advantage of short physical half-lives, cyclotron products can be obtained at very high specific activities and radionuclidic purity. However, because the cost of installing and operating a cyclotron is high, there are few of them and they are widely dispersed. The problem is therefore one of rapid transport of the short-lived nuclides, and in practice it has only been possible for centres with their own machine to use those nuclides with half-lives less than about 2 hours. Other centres, dependent on transport, have been limited to the use of nuclides with rather longer half-lives.

The very important radioactive isotopes of carbon, oxygen and nitrogen, which are of great significance biologically, have, with the exception of ^{14}C, very short half-lives and therefore can only be used with a cyclotron on site. Those used in clinical practice are listed in Table 5.4; they can all be produced in low-energy machines (12 MeV proton, 6 MeV deuteron). Such a 'baby cyclotron' machine is now in production in Switzerland (High Energy and Nuclear Equipment SA). It is a 'light-weight' cyclotron, weighing 7½ tonnes, and does not require an expensive, heavily shielded room. ^{11}C, ^{13}N and ^{15}O are all positron emitters and therefore have the associated 0.51 MeV annihilation γ-radiation; this property has been utilised in tomographic scanning. Some of the applications of these three nuclides are summarised in Table 5.5.

The cyclotron-produced nuclides with half-lives of 1 hour or more have a wider distribution. Table 5.6 shows these, together with their applications. The nuclide with probably the greatest potential is ^{123}I; this is because there are a large number of biologically important molecules which can be iodinated. Many of these are already in use labelled with ^{125}I and ^{131}I, but neither of these is ideal for imaging with a gamma camera, whereas ^{123}I has the ideal physical properties.

There are some cyclotron-produced generators which produce daughter-products with very short half-lives of seconds only. Two

Table 5.4 *Cyclotron-produced radioisotopes of carbon, nitrogen and oxygen used in clinical practice*

Element	Nuclide	Half-life (minutes)	Mode of decay	β^+-energy (MeV)	Photon energy (MeV)
Carbon	^{11}C	20.3	β^+	0.98	0.511 annihilation
Nitrogen	^{13}N	10.0	β^+	1.19	0.511 annihilation
Oxygen	^{15}O	2.07	β^+	1.7	0.511 annihilation

of these coming into use are the krypton-81m generator and the rubidium-82 generator. ^{81m}Kr has a half-life of 13 seconds and is formed by the decay of rubidium-81 (half-life 4.7 hours); ^{82}Rb has a half-life of 75 seconds and is formed by the decay of strontium-82 (half-life 25 days). The former has been used for cerebral blood-flow measurements, and the latter for myocardial imaging.

Table 5.5 *Medical applications of ^{11}C, ^{13}N and ^{15}O*

Nuclide	Chemical form	Applications
^{11}C	^{11}CO gas $^{11}CO_2$ gas	Lung function
	^{11}CO-labelled red cells	Measurement of red cell volume; imaging of blood pool
	[^{11}C] palmitic acid	Imaging of myocardial infarcts
	^{11}C-labelled psychotic drugs (e.g. [^{11}C] chlorpromazine)	Dynamic brain imaging
	[^{11}C] glucose	Imaging of brain metabolism
^{13}N	$^{13}N_2$ gas	Lung function
	$^{13}NH_3$	Investigation of blood perfusion in brain
^{15}O	$^{15}O_2$ gas ^{15}CO gas $^{15}CO_2$ gas $H_2{}^{15}O$	Lung function

Table 5.6 *Medical applications of cyclotron-produced radionuclides (other than ^{11}C, ^{13}N and ^{15}O)*

Nuclide	Half-life	Chemical form	Applications
^{123}I	13 hours	Iodide	Thyroid function
		Hippuran	Renography
		Rose Bengal	Liver function
		Hexadecenoic acid	Myocardial imaging
^{43}K ^{24}Na ^{77}Br	22 hours 21 hours 56 hours	Chloride Chloride Chloride	Electrolyte studies
^{18}F ^{87}Y	1.8 hours 1.3 hours	Fluoride Parent nuclide for ^{87m}Sr	Bone imaging (^{87m}Sr, $T_{\frac{1}{2}}$ 2.8 hours)
^{81}Rb	4.6 hours	Parent nuclide for ^{81m}Kr generator	Regional lung function (^{81m}Kr, $T_{\frac{1}{2}}$ 13 seconds)
^{111}In ^{67}Ga	2.8 days 78 hours	Bleomycin Citrate	Tumour localisation
^{52}Fe	8.3 hours	Citrate	Bone marrow imaging
^{127}Xe	36.4 days	Gas	Cerebral blood flow

The limitation on the use of cyclotron-produced nuclides is at present imposed by cost and availability. It is hoped that in the not too distant future this situation may improve.

Legislation

Council Directive of 1 June 1976

The treaty establishing the European Atomic Energy Commission (EAEC) prescribed that basic standards must be laid down for the protection of the health of the general public and workers against the dangers arising from ionising radiations, in order to enable each member state to make provisions by legislation to ensure compliance with the basic standards. On 1 June 1976, the Council of the European Communities approved the directive laying down revised basic safety standards (EC Council Directive, 1976). The directive is addressed to the member states; article 40 requires each member state to have put into effect the necessary measures to conform to the directive within a period of two years from the date of notification (i.e. by July 1978), and to inform the commission of the arrangements it has made to comply with the directive. At the time of going to press it is understood that a new directive is about to be issued, and that its implementation date will be July 1980.

The directive deals with two aspects of safety; it is mainly concerned with the limitation of radiation doses received by exposed workers and members of the public, but control of administration of radioactive substances is also required (article 5a). The latter aspect is dealt with here, the former will be dealt with in Chapter 11.

The directive requires that a system of prior authorisation must be applied in respect of the administration of radioactive substances to persons for the purposes of treatment, diagnosis or research. In this context the EAEC defines a radioactive substance as any substance that contains one or more radionuclides of which the activity or concentration cannot be disregarded as far as radiation protection is concerned.

Regulations in the UK

Administration. In the UK the Secretary of State has decided to implement article 5a using powers under the Medicines Act 1968. This required regulations to be made under section 60 of the act, which are cited as The Medicines (Administration of Radioactive Substances) Regulations 1978, and a supporting order under section 104 of the act, which is cited as The Medicines (Radioactive Substances) Order 1978. The order is required to bring administration of radiopharmaceuticals to volunteers within the control of the Regulations.

The Regulations 1978 require that no person shall either administer to any human being a radiopharmaceutical, or perform in-vivo activation analysis unless he is a practitioner holding a certificate granted for that purpose under the Regulations, or a person acting in accordance with the directions of such a practitioner. It will be an offence to administer a radiopharmaceutical or to perform in-vivo activation analysis without an appropriate certificate. Certificates of authorisation will be granted by the Secretary of State as advised by the Administration of Radioactive Substances Advisory Committee (ARSAC). This committee also has a non-statutory function, that of giving informal guidance on the use of radiopharmaceuticals in clinical medicine and research. The Health Ministers are responsible for enforcing the Medicines Act and associated Regulations. This is likely to be achieved by routine examination of authorisation certificates and stock control records to see that amounts administered are in line with the recommendations, and that proper records are being kept.

Manufacture. The Medicines Act 1968 requires that manufacturers of pharmaceuticals must hold a licence for each product on the market, and radiopharmaceuticals are included in this. New radiopharmaceuticals being supplied by a manufacturer for clinical trials must be covered by a clinical trial certificate, which may be obtained from the licensing authority. The latter is advised by the Committee on Safety of Medicines, and another committee, to be called the Committee on Radiation from Radioactive Medicinal Products, will be set up to advise on the radiation aspects of any substance for human use.

The position with respect to the preparation of radiopharmaceuticals on hospital premises is less clearly defined; obviously this preparation must conform with standards imposed by the Medicines Act, and departments responsible for the preparations are subject to inspection by the Medicines Inspectorate, a branch of the Medicines Division. To date there is no clear directive from the Medicines Division regarding the pharmaceutical facilities required, but outline guidance on good radiopharmaceutical manufacturing practice is being developed by the Medicines Inspectorate.

Appendix. Samples of Master Control Documents for radiopharmaceutical preparations

Procedure for use of clean room and laminar flow cabinet

(1) Switch on fan which draws filtered air from the corridor into the laboratory.
(2) The window must be kept *closed* at all times.
(3) Open the front panel of the laminar flow panel and switch fan on.
(4) The fan should be on for at least 15 minutes before any aseptic procedure is carried out. During this time all surfaces within the cabinet should be cleaned with 70% methylated spirits.
(5) Entry to the 'hot' laboratory must be from the sliding door to laboratory 1. This door must be kept closed whenever possible; the door to the corridor must be kept locked at all times.
(6) Before commencing any aseptic procedure, hands must be thoroughly washed in Hibitane, dried, and Triflex gloves worn.
(7) Meticulous attention must be paid to the maintenance of sterility, and the instructions contained in the master document for each procedure followed exactly. There must be no equipment or materials (e.g. syringes, needles, syringe containers) within the laminar flow cabinet, except those in immediate use.
(8) At the end of the day's work swab the inner surfaces of the cabinet with 70% methylated spirits, switch off the fan and light and close the front panel. Switch off the intake fan from corridor.
(9) Settle plates, which are kept in the refrigerator, must be placed, one at the rear of the cabinet on the right, the other at the front on the left, weekly, preferably on Wednesday mornings, and exposed for 1 hour. These should then be taken to the quality control laboratory in the pharmacy for incubation; a record of these tests must be kept in the book provided.
(10) All benches, walls (below the shelves), sinks, etc. must be cleaned thoroughly with 70% methylated spirits, weekly, preferably on a Friday. The person must record that this has been carried out, in the book provided.

Sterilisation procedures

1. *Radioactive solutions which are heat stable, and are of reasonably long half-life*
   These must be autoclaved either:
   (i) in the autoclave for 20 minutes, after the thermometer has reached 120 °C;
   (ii) in the pressure cooker for 45 minutes at 10 lb pressure (NB one of the perforated baskets must be used).
   In either case a Browne's tube (Black Spot), in a similar container, must be put in with each batch and the colour change checked before removing the solutions as sterile.
   Multi-dose vials. After removing activity from a multi-dose vial, the latter must be re-sterilised if it is going to be used again. This must be carried out the same half day.

2. *Glassware etc.*
   (i) Glassware must be placed in closed canisters and heated in the oven for 1 hour at 160 °C. A Browne's tube (Green Spot), in a canister, must be put in the oven with each batch, and the colour change checked before removing as sterile.
   (ii) Closed glass bottles, tubes, etc. (especially those with rubber caps, for which dry sterilisation is unsuitable) may be sterilised in the autoclave for 20 minutes after the thermometer has reached 120 °C. These must contain a small quantity of liquid, e.g. 0.1 ml water, for injection.

3. *Instruments in direct contact with steam*
   These must be sterilised in the autoclave for 10 minutes after the thermometer has reached 120 °C, or in boiling water, in the pressure cooker, for 30 minutes.

4. *Radioactive solutions which are not heat stable, and/or have short half-lives, or are required for use without delay*

^{131}I-labelled albumin ^{125}I-labelled albumin	see preparation of ^{131}I (or ^{125}I) HSA doses for renograms
^{99m}Tc as pertechnetate	(half-life of 6 hours)
^{113m}In in ionic form	(half-life of 1.67 hours)

   These must be sterilised by Millipore filtration using millex filter type no. SL65 025 05, pore size 0.22 μm.
   A sample (0.5 ml) must be sent to the Bacteriology Department for sterility testing.

5. *Radioactive solutions which are not heat stable, and/or have short half-lives, and contain particle suspension which are too large for Millipore filtration*
   e.g. ^{99m}Tc as macroaggregated HSA (half-life 6 hours)
   ^{51}Cr as labelled red cells
   These must be prepared under strictly sterile conditions. A sample of MAA (0.5 ml) must always be sent to Bacteriology for sterility testing. A sample of labelled red cells (0.5 ml) must be sent to Bacteriology for sterility testing, from every third preparation.

6. *^{99m}Tc weekly checks*
   Samples (0.5 ml) from the following should be sent to Bacteriology for sterility testing:
   6.1. One ^{99m}Tc-labelled antimony sulphide colloid sample, labelled to include the day of its preparation.
   6.2. One ^{99m}Tc-labelled EHDP sample, labelled to include the day of its preparation.
   6.3. The multi-dose eluate vial; the sample for testing must be taken at the end of the day (preferably on Friday) after all the doses for that day have been withdrawn.
   6.4. The multi-dose eluate vial; the sample for testing must be taken on Fridays immediately after milking the column *before* the eluate has been autoclaved. This will check the sterility of the generator.

General rules
All sterilised material which is not being used immediately must bear a green label. This label must seal the outside of the canister or bottle as soon as it is taken out of the steriliser in a sterile condition, or has been put through a Millipore filter. Any canister, bottle or ampoule which does not have an unbroken green seal must be regarded as non-sterile and must not be used for intravenous injection. Labels giving details of the content of all radioactive solutions must be written out before they are sterilised. The labels must be placed in a clear position, either on the steriliser or on the bench immediately in front of the steriliser. They must be placed on the bottles as soon as they are taken out of the steriliser.

Administration of radioactive material. No radioactive material must be administered, by injection, orally, or by any other route, *without the label* (bearing details of the isotope and its activity) *being checked by a second person.* If the material is being administered by a doctor, he may be asked to check the label. If the material is being administered by one of the staff of the department, the check must be made by another of the staff. Each syringe containing a dispensed dose must be assayed and then placed in a separate tray (ready for injection), with the patient's name, date, type of test, isotope, activity and volume clearly stated on the label.

Preparation of ^{99m}Tc labelled colloid for liver scans

Dose for adult is 2 mCi ^{99m}Tc

NB All procedures to be carried out aseptically in the laminar flow cupboard.

(1) Place a sterile glass vial in a lead container and swab the top with methylated spirit.
(2) Add 5 ml of preformed antimony sulphide colloid to the sterile vial.
(3) Add 0.12 ml of sterile normal hydrochloric acid.
(4) Add 2.5 ml ^{99m}Tc as pertechnetate in isotonic saline as eluate from the column. (If less activity is required, less volume of ^{99m}Tc may be used, the volume being made up to 2.5 ml with isotonic saline) Label.
(5) Autoclave at 120 °C for 30 minutes.
(6) Remove from the autoclave and cool as quickly as possible.
(7) Add 1 ml 10% sodium acetate and mix well.
(8) Draw up the required dose and inspect visually. The material should be clear orange and particle free.
(9) Measure the dose in the dose calibrator.
(10) Send a small sample to Bacteriology for sterility testing.

Preparation of ^{99m}Tc-labelled HSA microspheres for lung scans

Kit: TCK-5, supplied from 'Sorin' by Eurotope Services Ltd; stored at room temperature.
Each vial contains 10 mg microspheres of human serum albumin (1 400 000 particles, 95% of which have a diameter between 12 and 36 μm) plus 0.9 mg stannous chloride.
Check expiry date has not been reached.

(1) Swab vial top after placing vial in lead shield.
(2) Add ^{99m}Tc in 5 ml normal saline.
(3) Invert carefully several times to suspend the microspheres.
(4) Label with the activity, date, volume and time.
(5) Place vial in lead pot in mechanical shaker and shake at position 4 for 15 minutes.
(6) Make up dose *immediately* prior to injection into patient,

shaking vial whilst drawing up dose to keep microspheres in suspension. Check in dose calibrator.

Adult dose 2 mCi

Child dose 0.03 ml mCi/kg

(7) Check syringe in dose calibrator after dose has been given.

(8) Send sample to Bacteriology for sterility testing.

References

BIR (1975). *Guidelines for the Preparation of Radiopharmaceuticals in Hospitals.* London: British Institute of Radiology.

HPA (1977). *The Hospital Preparation of Radiopharmaceuticals.* London: Hospital Physicists' Association, Radionuclide Topic Group.

IAEA (1971). *Radionuclide Generators.* Vienna: International Atomic Energy Agency.

IAEA (1973). *Radiopharmaceuticals and Labelled Compounds*, vols. 1 and 2. Vienna: International Atomic Energy Agency.

Medicines Act (1968). London: HMSO.

USAEC (1966). *Radioactive Pharmaceuticals*, ed. G.A. Andrews, R.M. Kniseley & H.W. Wagner. Oak Ridge USA: USAEC Division of Technical Information Extension.

Medicines (Radioactive Substances) Order 1978.

Medicines (Administration of Radiopharmaceuticals) Regulations 1978.

6. Investigations involving measurements on samples only

Introduction

These are the simplest of all investigations, but need to be carried out with meticulous attention to detail if results are to be reliable. They fall into three main categories: dilution techniques, metabolic and other studies involving only blood-clearance and excretion measurements, and in-vitro studies.

Dilution techniques are used mainly to determine the volumes of body fluids, and total exchangeable body contents of electrolytes. The radiopharmaceutical is used as a tracer, that it, it is presumed to distribute in a way identical to the substance under investigation but is not necessarily isotopic with the latter. It is introduced into the appropriate body compartment and, after sufficient time has elapsed for equilibrium to be reached, a sample is withdrawn. From the concentration of the tracer in the sample it is possible to calculate the volume in which the sample is distributed. For example, the red cell volume may be measured by re-injecting a patient's blood after labelling the red cells with ^{51}Cr or ^{99m}Tc, and taking a blood sample 5 minutes after injection. This and other dilution techniques will be considered in more detail later, together with an account of the implicit assumptions and the sources of error.

Metabolic studies require true tracer techniques. If the metabolism of an element is being studied the radionuclide must be isotopic with that element; for example radioactive iodine is used to study iodine metabolism by the thyroid gland and radioactive iron to study iron turnover. The tracer of a compound being studied is that compound radioisotopically labelled by substituting a radioactive isotope for one of its atoms. Many such studies are used to investigate the metabolism of trace elements and drugs; most of the latter can only be labelled with ^{14}C or ^{3}H, which restricts measurements to samples only, because both isotopes are low-energy β-emitters, and cannot be detected externally. An example is the study of the metabolism of phenytoin using [^{3}H]phenytoin. Another type of study is that which involves the measurement of the clearance of substances from the blood; for example the measurement of the rate of clearance of radioactively-labelled EDTA complexes is used to calculate the glomerular filtration rate.

In-vitro studies are those in which no radioactivity is administered to the patient, the test being carried out using only a blood sample taken from the patient. The test usually involves adding a radioactive component to the patient's plasma and measuring its distribution between two phases. These techniques are very specialised, and it is not proposed to describe them in this book; however, most of the arguments concerning accuracy that are presented here will apply.

Dilution techniques

The points regarding basic assumptions and accuracy are best made by reference to an example.

The measurement of red cell and plasma volumes

The red cells are labelled with ^{51}Cr or ^{99m}Tc, and the plasma with ^{125}I, according to the procedures laid down in the master documents. The labelled red cells are resuspended in the labelled plasma, the blood re-injected, and blood samples taken. Since the photopeak of ^{125}I is much lower than that of either ^{51}Cr or ^{99m}Tc the ^{125}I radioactive content of the plasma can be measured simultaneously with the ^{51}Cr or ^{99m}Tc content of the red cells, by counting the whole-blood samples in two different channels as described in Chapter 3. The detailed procedure is given below, together with the sources of error, but since the errors are the same for both red cell volume and plasma volume only those as applied to the former will be discussed.

Detailed procedure. Taking the labelled blood referred to above:

(1) Mix the blood thoroughly on a blood-mixer for at least 15 minutes.

(2) Take off a standard of 0.5 ml into a 1 ml syringe; weigh the loaded syringe. Discharge the contents into a 100 ml measuring flask and make up accurately to 100 ml with distilled water containing a small amount of carrier. Mix thoroughly. Take off, by pipette, an accurate 5 ml sample into a counting tube. Re-weigh the empty syringe and subtract this value from the weight of the loaded syringe to obtain the weight, S, of red cells used to prepare the standard.

(3) Take up the remainder of the thoroughly mixed labelled blood into a weighed 20 ml syringe. Re-weigh the loaded syringe and obtain the weight, D, of red cells in the syringe.

(4) Inject the labelled blood intravenously into the patient, taking care to collect any that is spilt on to swabs or tissues. Wash out the empty syringe, transferring the wash into a counting tube and place any other remaining labelled blood lost to injection, i.e. swabs etc., into another counting tube.

(5) Take 7 ml blood samples, using a different vein from that used for injection, at 5, 15 and 60 minutes after injection, and place in a heparinised tube. Mix the samples thoroughly for at least 15 minutes and measure the haematocrit of each sample using the microcapillary method. Three haematocrit tubes should be loaded for each sample, the tubes being inserted to different depths. The mean value is taken.
(6) Haemolyse the blood samples with saponin, again mix thoroughly, and transfer 5 ml of each to a counting tube.
(7) Set the channel windows for ^{125}I and ^{51}Cr and count the following in a well-shaped scintillation counter to give a 1% statistical accuracy (i.e. 10 000 counts): an empty counting tube to serve as background; the ^{51}Cr (or ^{99m}Tc) and ^{125}I standards prepared when the blood was labelled; the combined ^{51}Cr/^{125}I standard; the three blood samples; and the supernatant from the washed blood cells, the wash from the empty injection syringe and any contaminated swabs etc.
(8) Calculate the red cell volume as follows.

Calculations. If the total ^{51}Cr radioactivity of the red cells injected

$$= A\ \mu\text{Ci(Bq)}$$

and the ^{51}Cr radioactivity per millilitre of red cells in the venous blood sample

$$= a\ \mu\text{Ci ml}^{-1}\ (\text{Bq ml}^{-1})$$

then the red cell volume (RCV)

$$= A/a \text{ ml} \tag{6.1}$$

But if the ^{51}Cr radioactivity in the whole-blood sample

$$= x\ \mu\text{Ci ml}^{-1}\ (\text{Bq ml}^{-1})$$

the volume of the whole-blood sample

$$= v \text{ ml}$$

and the haematocrit

$$= H$$

then

$$a = x/vH\ \mu\text{Ci ml}^{-1}\ (\text{Bq ml}^{-1})$$

and

$$\text{RCV} = \frac{A}{x}\, v\, H \text{ ml} \qquad (6.2)$$

Similarly the plasma volume

$$\text{PV} = \frac{B}{y}\, v\, (1 - H) \text{ ml} \qquad (6.3)$$

where B = total ^{125}I radioactivity of the plasma injected
y = total ^{125}I radioactivity in the whole-blood sample.

The accuracy of the result will be dependent on the accuracy with which the values of A/x, B/y, v and H can be obtained, and also on the validity of the assumptions implicit in the above equations.

It should be noted that equation 6.1 contains two assumptions:

(1) That all the radioactivity injected is attached to the red cells, that is, the injection is radiochemically pure, and that it remains in the red cells.

(2) That all the red cells remain in the vascular compartment.

The first assumption is justified by washing the red cells before injection and measuring the activity in the supernatant. Two washings are usually sufficient to ensure that the activity in the supernatant is below 1% of the total injected, but it should always be checked. The second assumption is normally valid up to 1 hour after injection, but may be checked by taking three blood samples at 5, 15 and 60 minutes respectively; a correction can be made if necessary.

The method is clearly very simple, but it should be noted that the accuracy of the result is dependent on the accuracy with which v and H are measured, and on the accuracy with which the radioactivity in the blood sample can be related to the activity injected (equation 6.2). The latter (A/x) is not quite so straightforward as may appear. If the two could be measured directly, under the same geometry with the same equipment, the ratio would be the ratio of their count-rates; but this is not practicable. It is therefore necessary to prepare a standard (see Procedure section, item 2), which is a known fraction of the injected dose, and of the same volume as the blood sample, so that equation 6.2 becomes

$$\text{RCV} = \frac{\text{count-rate on standard}}{\text{count-rate on whole-blood sample}}\, F\, v\, H$$

$$= \frac{C_S}{C_B}\, F\, v\, H \text{ ml} \qquad (6.4)$$

where

$$F = \frac{\text{weight of red cells injected}}{\text{weight of red cells in standard}} = \frac{D}{S/20}$$

If it can be ensured that, at the time of injection, none of the patient's blood enters the injection syringe, and none of the injection is lost on swabs etc., then the weight of the red cells injected is simply the difference in the weights of the syringe before and after injection. In practice this is difficult to achieve, and a correction must be applied for any red cell radioactivity lost to injection (C_E) and collected on swabs, tissues, etc. (C_M). Weight of red cells not injected

$$= \frac{(C_E + C_M)}{C_S} S/20$$

Therefore weight of red cells injected

$$= D - \left[\frac{C_E + C_M}{C_S} \right] S/20$$

therefore

$$F = \frac{20D}{S} \left[1 - \frac{(C_E + C_M)}{C_S} \frac{S}{20D} \right]$$

$$= \frac{C_I}{C_S} \left[1 - \frac{(C_E + C_M)}{C_I} \right]$$

where

$$C_I = C_S \frac{20D}{S}$$

i.e. the equivalent count-rate on the weighed injection dose if it were counted under the same conditions.

Sources of error. The overall error in the RCV is a combination of the errors on $[1 - (C_E + C_M)/C_I]$, D, S, v, H, C_S and C_B. It should be noted that all the count-rates are corrected for background, and dead-time losses if applicable, and the errors apply to the corrected count-rates. In this study the sample count-rates will be very high compared with background so that if at least 10 000 counts are taken the coefficient of variation will be 1% or better. D and S are both differences of two weighed quantities; accepting that the accuracy of weighing is probably to within 1 mg, in order to achieve 1% accuracy the weight difference should not be less than about 200 mg. The volume v should be within 1% with good pipetting technique; the coefficient of variation on the weighing and pipetting of each technician should previously have been determined. The haematocrit, even when great care is taken, is probably not accurate to within less than 2%. The most difficult to assess is the error on $[1 - (C_E + C_M)/C_I]$; the error on $(C_E + C_M)/C_I$ may be appreciable, because although the actual counts can be obtained to an accuracy of 1% by taking 10 000 counts, there will be other errors, due to differences in counting geometry and possibly due to radioactivity which is lost. If, however, the latter is kept small so that $(C_E + C_M)/C_I$ is, for example, less than 0.05, even if the error on it is as much as 20%, the error on $[1 - (C_E + C_M)/C_I]$ will be small. If $(C_E + C_M)/C_I$ is equal to 0.05 and has an error of 20%, the value of $[1 - (C_E + C_M)/C_I]$ will be 0.95 ± 0.01. It seems reasonable, therefore, to assume an error of about 1%. From the theory of errors (Chapter 4) the square of the overall percentage error E_{RCV} is given by the sum of the squares of the percentage errors of each of the experimental values, i.e.

$$E_{RCV}{}^2 = 1^2 + 1^2 + 1^2 + 1^2 + 1^2 + 1^2 + 2^2$$

$$E^2{}_{RCV} = 10$$

therefore

$$E_{RCV} \approx 3\%$$

In order to obtain the result to within ± 6% with a 95% level of confidence, it is necessary to keep the individual errors to those quoted above. It is evident, therefore, that there must be meticulous attention to detail throughout.

The measurement of electrolytes

When measurements of electrolytes are made, the method is based on the assumption that the injected labelled electrolyte equilibrates with the isotopic inactive body electrolyte, so that the ratio of labelled to total electrolyte is constant throughout the body. For example, if ^{43}K is injected intravenously, it is in equilibrium with the body potassium by 24 hours. If a blood sample is taken at 24 hours the volume of distribution of the ^{43}K can be calculated in exactly the same way as for the RCV, after allowing a correction of about 3% for ^{43}K excreted during the 24 hours. It should be appreciated that this volume of distribution, often referred to as the potassium space, has no physical meaning but is a useful physical concept. It is the hypothetical volume in which the potassium would be distributed if the concentration throughout were the same as the plasma concentration, and we know that this is not so. However, the total serum potassium can be measured by photometric methods, in moles per litre of plasma, and by multiplying that value by the value, in litres, of the potassium space, the value of the total exchangeable potassium is obtained. The latter is rather less than the total body potassium, because it includes only that potassium with which the ^{43}K is in equilibrium.

Studies involving the measurement of blood clearance

This type of study may simply aim at obtaining a graph of blood activity against time, with a view to fitting a mono- or multi-exponential curve or an empirical formula, or it may aim at quantitating the blood-clearance rate, in millilitres per minute. The latter is only a useful concept; it expresses the amount of a substance cleared per minute as the volume of blood which would be completely cleared if the substance were removed from that volume only and its concentration elsewhere were unchanged. The principles are best explained by example.

The measurement of glomerular filtration rate (GFR)

Many substances have been used for the measurement of GFR, the requirement being a substance which is cleared from the blood by free filtration at the glomerulus. ^{51}Cr-labelled EDTA has been found satisfactory, and a dose of 100 μCi (3.7 MBq) may be injected intravenously. The plasma clearance curve is obtained by taking blood samples at different times, and plotting the plasma activity against time. Although at first multi-exponential, the curve becomes mono-exponential after equilibrium is reached. Nimmon *et al.* (1974) have shown that using blood samples obtained at 3, 4, 5 and 6 hours, a mono-exponential curve may be fitted, and the results correlate well with the more rigorous method of using the whole area under the plasma clearance curve. The mono-exponential plasma-clearance curve may be represented by the equation

$$p = a_0 e^{-a_1 t} \qquad (6.5)$$

where p = plasma activity concentration in μCi ml^{-1} (MBq ml^{-1})
a_0 = plasma activity concentration obtained by extrapolation of the curve to zero time

a_1 = slope of the exponential in minutes^{-1}

The clearance rate, C, is calculated from the formula

$$C = \frac{D}{a_0/a_1} \text{ ml per minute} \tag{6.6}$$

where D = dose in μCi (MBq).

It will be evident that the same meticulous care is required in the preparation and measurement of the dose, standard, and plasma samples, since the same errors apply to D as in the RCV measurement. In addition there will be an error in the fitting of the mono-exponential, giving rise to errors on a_0 and a_1. The errors on a_0 and a_1 can be calculated if the method of least squares fit is used. The calculation is lengthy and requires a small computer program. Nimmon *et al.* (1974) have developed a program which uses a weighted least squares fit to take into account the statistical counting error and an estimated sampling error of 1% on each plasma sample, calculates the errors on a_0 and a_1, and then computes the overall error on C (E_C) from the errors on D, a_0 and a_1.

References

Nimmon, C.C., McAlister, J.M., Hickson, B. & Cattell, W.R. (1974). Study of the post-equilibrium slope approximation in the calculation of glomerular filtration rate using the ^{51}Cr-EDTA single injection technique. In *Dynamic Studies with Radioisotopes in Medicine*, vol. 1, pp. 249–56. Vienna: International Atomic Energy Agency.

7. Static radionuclide emission imaging

Introduction

The first imaging method used in medical diagnosis was the well-established one of radiology, which dates from the turn of the century and now includes sophisticated techniques such as tomography, neuroradiology and angiocardiography. Much later came the use of internally administered radionuclides, which could be located externally by detecting the radiation. This technique is referred to rather loosely in the nuclear medicine world as imaging. The first automatic rectilinear scanners were being built in 1950 and the first gamma camera was built in 1952. Rectilinear scanners were commercially available in 1959, and gamma cameras in 1964; the last two decades have seen great progress in instrumentation, and fast sophisticated equipment with data logging and data processing facilities and tomographic attachments is now available. In 1972 a new form of imaging was developed by EMI (Hounsfield, 1973), which is commonly known as computerised tomographic scanning (CT). More exactly it should be referred to as transmission computerised axial tomography (TCAT) to distinguish it from radionuclide tomography, which is emission computerised axial tomography (ECAT) (Kuhl & Edwards, 1963). The fourth imaging method is ultrasound; ultrasound is not new, but the much more sophisticated grey-scale techniques have given great impetus to its use, and it is now widely accepted as a valuable addition to diagnostic methods (Lunt, 1978). Two other techniques should also be mentioned. These are infra-red thermography and nuclear magnetic resonance. There is now a trend towards thinking in terms of 'Imaging departments' which include all these techniques, and to aim at a logical sequence of imaging investigations. The techniques are to some extent complementary since they do not look at the subject under investigation in the same way.

Conventional radiology

This demonstrates differences in X-radiation transmission due to differences in density and atomic number, at any moment in time; it has very sharp spatial resolution. The use of contrast media enables various organs to be defined and even the vascular system or lymphatic system to be visualised in great detail, but the latter are traumatic investigations not without hazard. Tomographic techniques are also used; these give greater sensitivity of detection because any density difference is related to the thickness in only a slice of tissue, and not to the whole-body thickness.

Transmission computerised axial tomography (TCAT)
This has great advantages over conventional radiology in the specialist areas. Firstly, it has much better density differentiation and can detect differences in tissue density of 0.5%. This is partly due to the tomographic effect but also to the use of scintillation detectors to detect the transmitted radiation and to the use of computer techniques to analyse and display the data. The second advantage is that it is an atraumatic technique; contrast material, if used, is injected intravenously. Compared with conventional radiology, the spatial resolution is less sharp.

Radionuclide imaging
This differs in one important aspect from the above two methods, in that it gives information about function. When radiopharmaceuticals are injected which are specifically taken up by an organ, a lack of uptake, or delay in uptake or excretion, denotes loss of function in the organ or part of the organ. In dynamic techniques it is possible to display functional images, as will be explained later. Radionuclide methods also have the great advantage of being atraumatic, and in general, with the advent of short-lived radiopharmaceuticals, they give rise to lower radiation doses than the two techniques described above. It must be remembered, though, that there is always some whole-body radiation, whereas with the two X-ray methods the radiation is restricted to the area under investigation. Tomographic techniques (ECAT) have been developed to give greater sensitivity of detection.

Ultrasound
These investigations demonstrate other properties of the tissue, for the reflection of ultrasound is dependent on back-scatter and absorption, and reflections thus occur when there are discontinuities of viscosity and elasticity as well as of density.

Infra-red thermography
This technique (Woodrough, 1979) is concerned with measuring skin temperature by imaging the emitted infra-red radiation. The detector output can be calibrated in terms of temperature. Since skin temperature is closely related to blood flow in superficial vessels, infra-red thermography has many applications to vascular disease and also provides useful information in a number of other clinical situations. Malignant tumours, for example, are associated with an increased vascularity and, being metabolically active, can

cause a considerable rise in the temperature of the blood which flows from the tumour.

Nuclear magnetic resonance
NMR is a technique which causes excitation of the protons in a sample by placing it in a magnetic field; their return to equilibrium is characterised by the spin-lattice relaxation times, which have been found to be longer for tumours than for normal tissue. The use of this technique for imaging is still in the experimental stage.

It is evident from the above descriptions that the techniques must be regarded as to some extent complementary. However, in many cases the first investigation may provide the information required and the choice of that investigation will be governed by, apart from clinical judgement, the ease and speed with which it can be carried out, and its cost. In this context radionuclide imaging has an established role to play.

Radionuclide imaging

The essential problem of radionuclide imaging is to reconstruct the distribution of an administered radionuclide within the body by means of external detection of the radiation, and to detect abnormalities which show as a deviation from the accepted normal distribution. The deviation may be an area either of increased activity or of reduced activity. It is assumed that the distribution of the radionuclide is the same as that of the administered radiopharmaceutical; the factors which may affect this basic assumption are discussed in Chapter 6.

The whole imaging process is shown in Fig. 7.1 (Mallard, 1972). It is divided into four components: collimator, detector, data transfer and display. The collimator selects the required γ-rays which proceed from the object, and allows only these through to the detector. The detector converts some of the γ-ray photons to, usually, electrical pulses, which the data transfer device transmits to the display system. It is also necessary for the data transfer system to transmit positional information with regard to the origin of each γ-ray photon. In a rectilinear scanner the display system is made to move in synchronism with the detector, which 'looks' only at the thin pencil of tissue over which it is temporarily centred. In a stationary detector, such as a camera, the detector 'looks' at the whole field of view, and records all the photons simultaneously; the positional information is obtained by electronic means. The display unit produces a map of the count-rate, which represents the distribution of radioactivity in the body. This map is referred to as the image, and the accuracy with which it reflects the object, that is the true distribution, is dependent on many factors.

Each component of the imaging system will produce some degradation of the image. The design of imaging equipment and the technique of imaging are both aimed at producing an image with minimum degradation. The factors which affect the quality of an image are: the sensitivity, resolution and distortion of the imaging system; the quantum statistics of the source; and the scattering and absorption of the radiation emitted by the source. The problem of scattering and absorption may be appreciated by drawing an analogy with the perception of objects by the eye, which is achieved by light waves or photons proceeding from an object to the eye and forming an image on the retina. Under normal daylight conditions light travels in approximately straight lines and there is little scattering or absorption of light in air; the image is thus a good reproduction of the object. However, under foggy conditions the light is scattered by particles of water vapour in the air and does not travel in straight lines, so that a blurred image is produced, a phenomenon with which we are all familiar. Filters such as sunglasses may be used to absorb some of the light reaching the eye in brilliant sunshine, but on going indoors to a poorly illuminated room the same filter reduces the number of

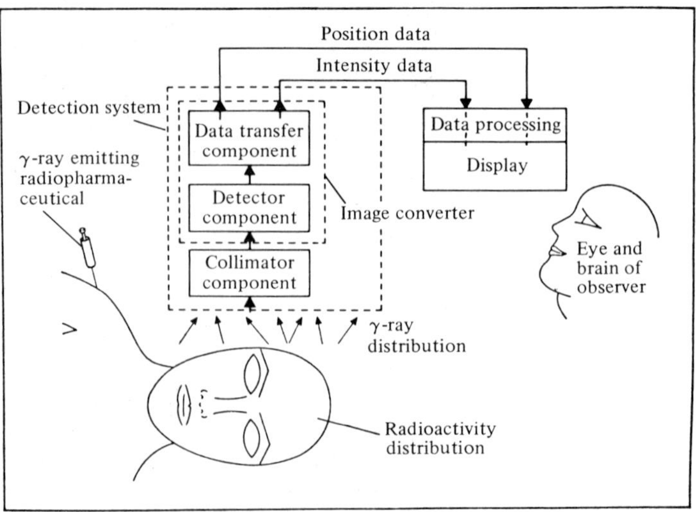

Fig. 7.1. Schematic diagram of the whole imaging process. (Reproduced from Mallard (1972), by kind permission of the publishers Karger and University Park Press.)

photons reaching the eye to a point where it is difficult to see.

Both the quantum statistics of the source and the sensitivity of the system affect the number of photons which produce the image. It has been shown by Rose (1957) that a good-quality television picture requires 10^7 photons, and he has demonstrated the improvement of the quality of the picture as the number of photons is increased from 3×10^3 to 2.8×10^7 (Fig. 7.2). Resolution is determined by the accuracy with which the origin of a γ-ray photon in the radioactive source can be reproduced, and this is governed by the scattering of the radiation, by the collimation, and by the transfer device which transmits the spatial information. The problems are rather different for rectilinear scanners and stationary detectors, and these will be considered separately, but first it is necessary to define sensitivity and resolution, and to discuss general problems of collimation.

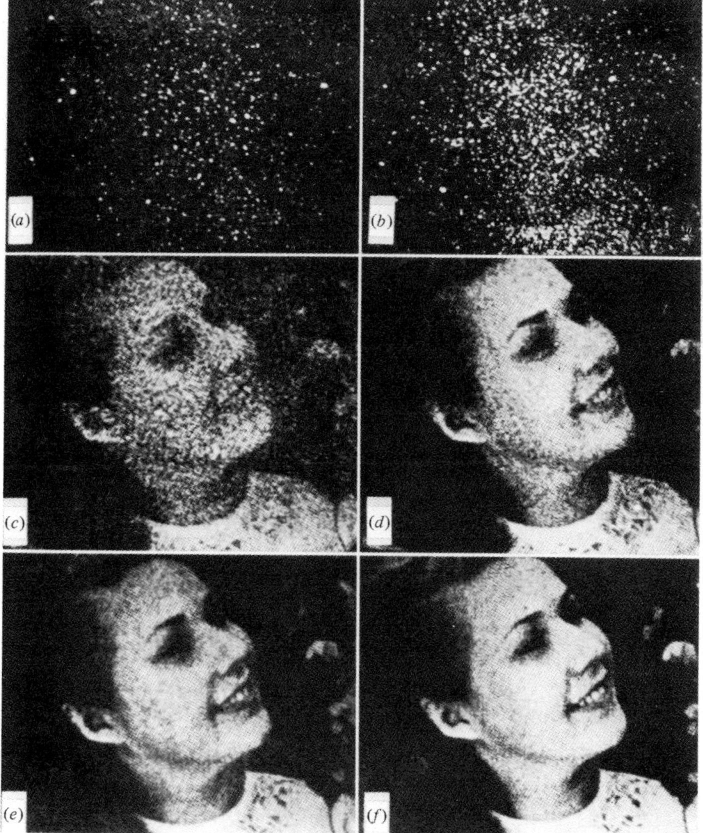

Fig. 7.2. Dependence of picture quality on number of incident photons. Note the improvement of the picture as the number of photons increases from 3×10^3 in (*a*) to 2.8×10^7 in (*e*). (Reproduced from Rose (1972), by kind permission of the publishers Academic Press.)

In order to facilitate comparisons between different pieces of imaging equipment, definitions and test conditions have been laid down in the IEC draft document 62C (1977); much information used in this was derived from a report to the International Commission on Radiation Units and Measurements (MacIntyre *et al.*, 1969).

Sensitivity

The sensitivity of an imaging system is that characteristic which expresses the number of photons counted by the detection system in terms of the number of photons emitted from the radioactive source to which the system is exposed. It will obviously be dependent on the geometry of the source with respect to the detector. Four types of sensitivity, namely point, line, plane and volume, have been used for sensitivity measurement; each gives a characteristic set of sensitivity values.

The IEC draft document specifies that, for the purposes of assessing imaging equipment, sensitivity shall be characterised by plane sensitivity, defined as follows: 'With a specified collimator and PHA window [plane sensitivity is] the ratio of the count-rate of the detector head to the activity (of a specified nuclide) per unit area of a standard plane source, placed in air perpendicular to, and centred on, the collimator axis at a specified distance Z from the collimator front face.' In the case of a focussed collimator the source is to be placed in the effective focal plane, and otherwise at a distance of 100 mm from the collimator face (Fig. 7.3). The source is to be a radioactive solution in a cuvette of Lucite with parallel sides; the dimensions of the cuvette are specified. The activity of the source should be known to an accuracy better than ± 5%. The sensitivity is then expressed as counts per second per microcurie (or megabecquerel) per square centimetre, and will hold for the radionuclide measured using a specified channel width. The sensitivity will, of course, vary with the collimator.

Resolution

Spatial resolution can be defined qualitatively as the capability of a system to distinguish fine detail in the image, and phantoms have been designed to test this. A quantitative definition introduces the concept of a line spread function (LSF). This is used in the IEC document and is defined as 'The function $L(X)$ giving some measured quantity, for example count-rate, as a function of the X-coordinate, when a line source is placed in a plane perpendicular to the collimator axis, parallel with the Y-axis and at a specified distance Z from the collimator face' (Fig. 7.4). A line source is defined as a radioactive solution in a tube of internal

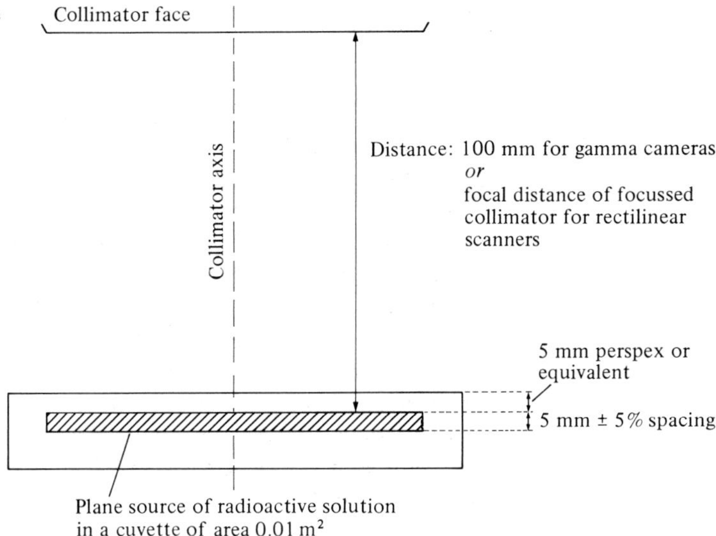

Fig. 7.3. Set-up for the measurement of plane sensitivity.

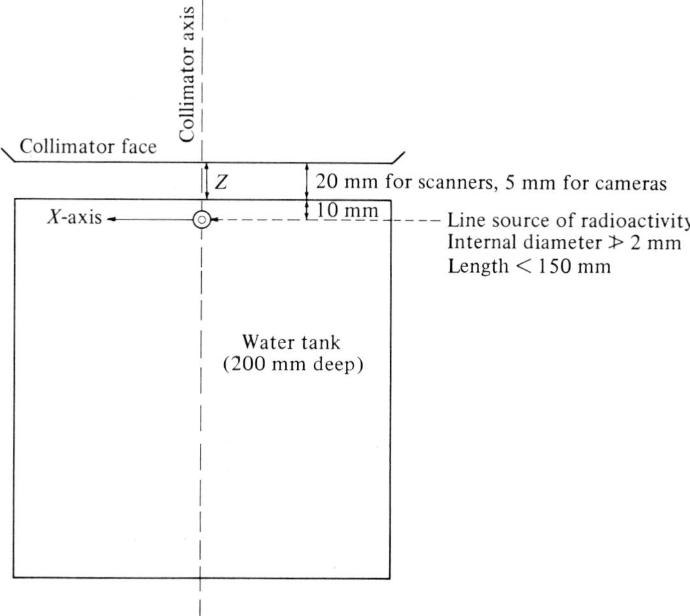

Fig. 7.4. Set-up for the measurement of line spread function.

diameter less than 2 mm and of specified length. The LSF is obtained by measuring the count-rate at various distances from the source, along the X-axis, that is perpendicular to and in the same plane as the line source. Measurements should preferably be continued until the count-rate is reduced to 1% of the maximum value. A linear plot of the count-rate against x gives the LSF (Fig. 7.5). From this curve it is possible to obtain the full-width-at-half-maximum (FWHM), which is defined as the distance along the X-axis between the points where the LSF has half its maximum value. The FWHM may be used as an index of resolution: two parallel and equal line sources separated by the FWHM should just be resolved. The LSF is to be measured in a water phantom for a set of planes 10 or 20 mm apart, starting in a plane with the centre of the source at 30 mm from the collimator face for a scanner (20 mm for a camera) and continuing until the value of the counts on the collimator axis is less than 10% of its maximum value. It will be evident that the LSF curve broadens appreciably at increased depths, due to the effect of scattered radiation.

A set of LSF curves contains all the information necessary to describe completely the spatial resolution of a detection system. A more complete expression of the information is the modular transfer function (MTF), which is the Fourier transform of the LSF (MacIntyre *et al.*, 1969).

Fig. 7.5. Line spread function of rectilinear scanner.

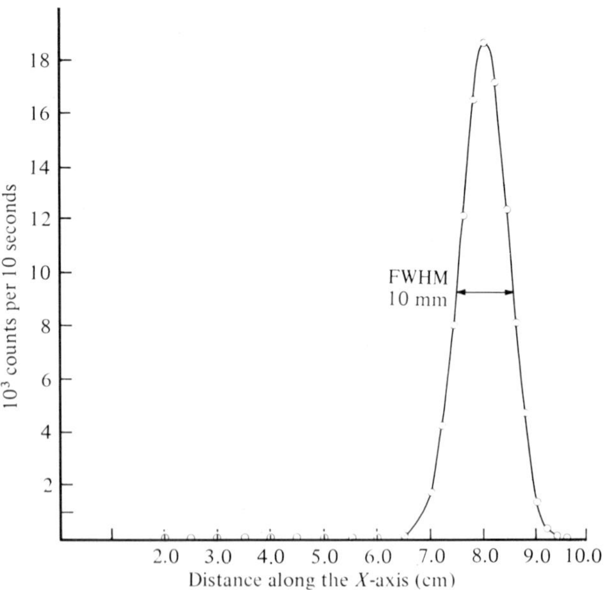

Collimation

A gamma camera, as will be explained later, has intrinsic resolution, but collimation is needed to direct the γ-rays proceeding from a three-dimensional object and to reduce the scattered radiation that reaches the crystal. The resolution of a rectilinear scanner is entirely dependent on collimation. The collimator performs a function somewhat analogous to a lens in a camera. However, as γ-rays cannot easily be refracted, the collimator functions only by absorbing radiation from unwanted directions and areas; it may be defined as a block of radiation-attenuating material with one or more apertures that limit the angular spread of the radiation which can reach the radiation detector assembly. The apertures and the material separating them are referred to as holes and septa respectively.

Positioning of patient

Positioning is of great importance in radionuclide imaging, as in all imaging techniques. It is essential to ensure that true anterior, posterior, or lateral views are obtained, since interpretation is based on recognition of a normal pattern, and of deviations from that pattern, and also sometimes on a lack of symmetry. Since anatomical detail is not clearly defined, it is not always possible to distinguish between a result caused by poor positioning and one caused by a true abnormality. In addition, it is often necessary to show anatomical landmarks on the image, and sometimes it is helpful to take a radiograph with the patient in the same position, using lead markers to correlate points on the radionuclide image with those on the radiograph.

Rectilinear scanners

A rectilinear scanner, as stated earlier, is essentially a device in which the detector sees only the radiation from the thin pencil of tissue over which it is temporarily centred. This is achieved by the use of collimators. The detector is moved automatically over the whole area of interest, and the display unit, which is made to move in synchronism with the detector, builds up a picture of the radiation detected in that area. It should be noted that at each point the detector looks at the whole depth of tissue, so that a two-dimensional image is formed of a three-dimensional object. Specialised scanners have been designed to provide tomographic facilities for section scanning (see the section on tomography, p. 121).

Fig. 7.6. (*a*) Modern dual-detector rectilinear scanner. (Photograph provided by Laboratory Impex Ltd (Selo).) (*b*) Colour display system of above. (Photograph provided by Laboratory Impex Ltd (Selo).)

(*a*)

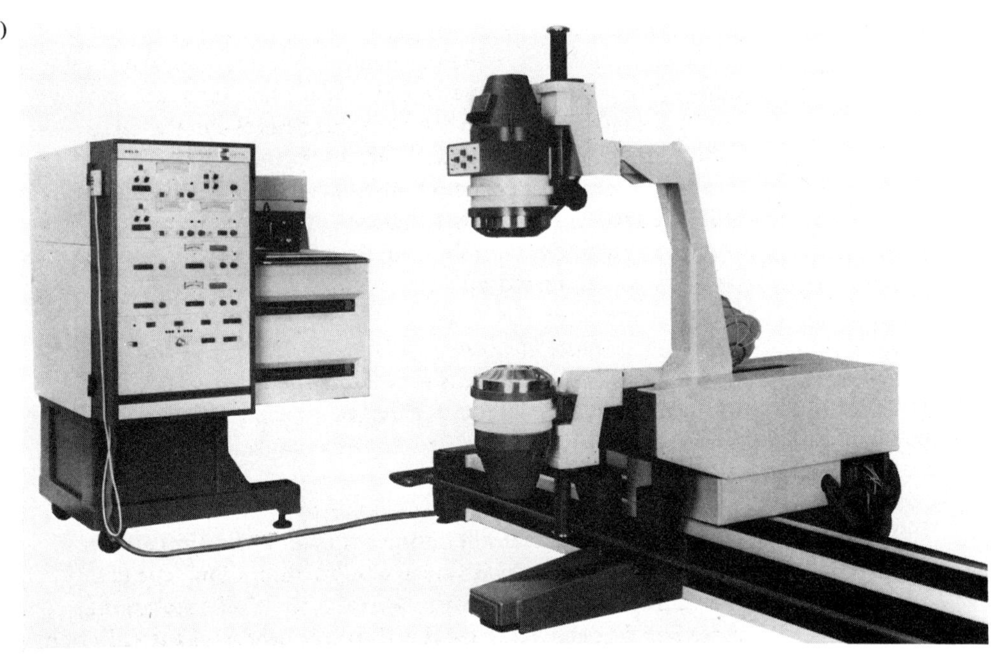

(*b*)

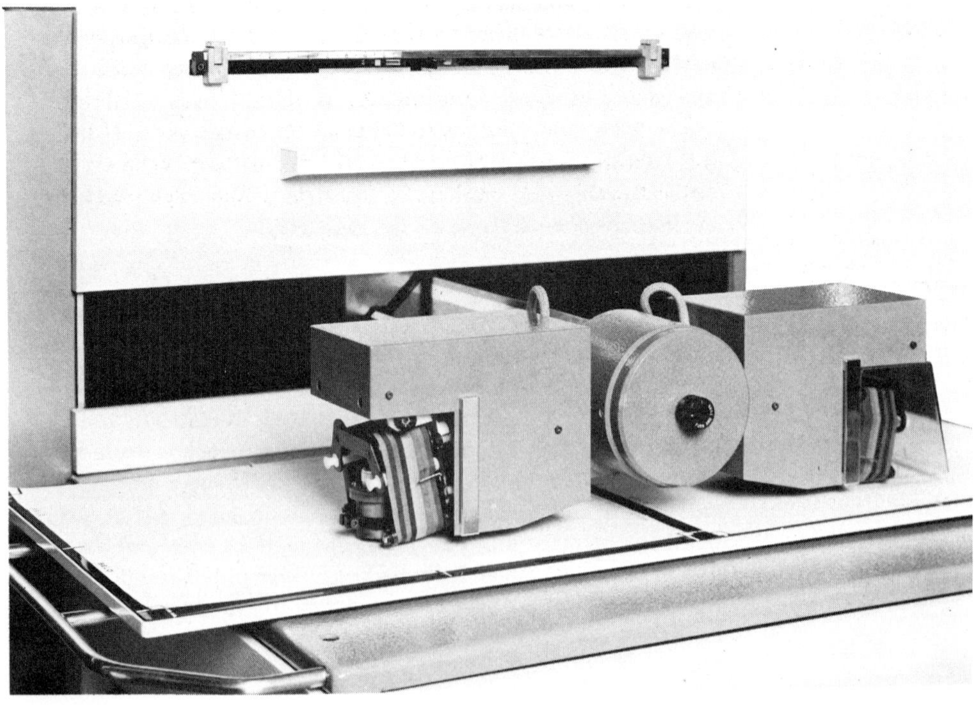

A photograph of a modern dual detector rectilinear scanner is shown in Fig. 7.6(*a*), and a photograph of the colour display system in (*b*). It can be seen from Fig. 7.6(*a*) that the transfer of positional information is by simple mechanical coupling; the detector and the display system are at opposite ends of a rigid horizontal beam and therefore always move in synchronism. In other systems the coupling is achieved by electronic means.

Factors which need to be considered when using a rectilinear scanner are considered below.

Collimation, sensitivity and resolution

The detector and its associated electronic equipment are as described in the section on NaI scintillation counters in Chapter 3 (p. 24) although the NaI crystal is usually larger than in sample counters to increase sensitivity.

The type of collimator that is almost invariably used with a rectilinear scanner is the focussed collimator, in which all the holes are tapered and all converge to the same point, the geometrical focus, on the collimator axis (Fig. 7.7*a*). Ideally, the septa should be sufficiently thick, for the energy of the radiation being used, to prevent septal penetration, and this can readily be achieved with low-energy γ-radiation. Under these conditions only the collimated primary radiation (plus some scattered radiation which arises in the collimator itself) will reach the detector.

The performance of a collimator may be assessed in several ways, including the measurement of LSF described earlier. Another method is to calculate, or measure, the response of the

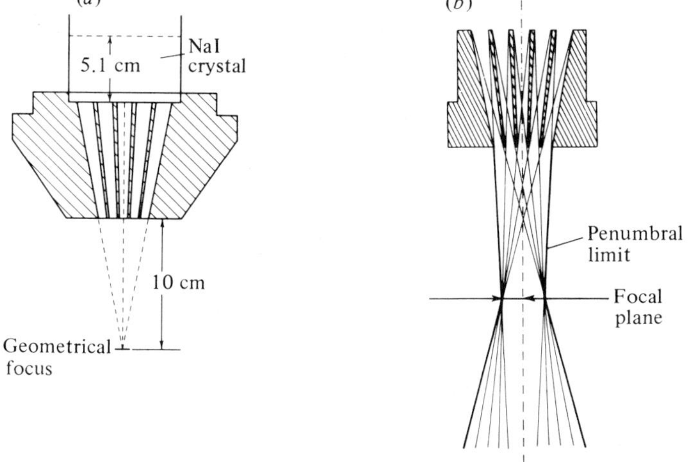

Fig. 7.7. Typical multi-hole focussed collimator, (*a*) showing geometrical focus and (*b*) showing superimposed penumbra in the focal plane. (Reprinted from G. Hine (ed.) (1967), *Instrumentation in Nuclear Medicine*, vol. 1, by kind permission of the publishers, Academic Press.)

collimator–detector system to a point source of radioactivity at various distances, that is obtain point-source isoresponse curves. Such curves may be calculated from purely geometrical considerations by first calculating the response due to a single collimator hole, and then summing for all holes; these calculated curves are very similar to experimental curves obtained in air, if there is no septal penetration. Fig. 7.7(*b*) shows the superimposed penumbra due to the multiple holes, at the geometrical focus.

Experimental point-source isoresponse curves may be obtained by taking a point source of the radionuclide under investigation and moving it in a plane perpendicular to the collimator axis; this can be done at various depths. After finding the point of maximum response, which is the focus, and will obviously be on the axis of the collimator, it is possible to interpolate the measurements to produce lines of equal response, e.g. 90%, 80%, etc. of the maximum. Since collimators are symmetrical, a response curve is only required in one plane through the axis. Such response curves in air are normally provided for each collimator by the manufacturer. Of greater practical importance is the collimator response to sources in a tissue-equivalent scattering medium, and to establish this it is necessary to have response curves to a point source in water or other tissue-equivalent material. This is very laborious unless some automation is available, but it is worth doing.

Fig. 7.8(*a*) and (*b*) show typical collimator isoresponse curves for a collimator of nominal focus 10 cm due to a point source of ^{131}I in air and in water. The resolution, defined as the FWHM at the focus, is 1.5 cm in air and 1.6 cm in water. The focal distance in air is 9 cm and in water, with an air gap of 2.5 cm, is 6 cm. Fig. 7.8(*c*) shows the isoresponse curves for the summed output of two opposing detectors, and demonstrates a fairly uniform response (80%–100%) throughout a 20 cm water tank.

It will be seen that with the single detectors, although the response in water is greater than 80% for a source at depths between 0.5 cm and 8 cm, it falls off to less than 50% at depths greater than 10 cm. This means that the two-dimensional image will contain more data from the planes of high response than from those of low response. If a short-focus collimator is used it will produce a partial tomographic effect by selecting the plane at the focus. This can be useful in imaging small lesions and is particularly useful if these are superficial.

A colour representation or photodisplay of collimator response in air or water may easily be obtained by preparing a line radioactive source and placing it at an angle of 45 degrees to the collimator axis, and scanning it in the conventional way (Fig. 7.9).

Even if the full response curves are not obtained, it is important to know the central-axis depth response in order to operate the equipment intelligently, and to interpret the results. Central-axis depth response curves for ^{99m}Tc in water are given in Fig. 7.10, for air gaps of 2.5 cm, 5.0 cm and 7.5 cm, showing how it is possible to obtain some degree of focussing on to an organ of interest. As shown in Fig. 7.8(*c*), with two detectors, one anterior and one posterior, it is possible to obtain a fairly uniform response throughout the whole depth by summing the outputs of the two detectors; the response curves for a ^{99m}Tc source in a 20 cm deep water tank obtained with two detectors in parallel is shown in Fig. 7.11. A uniform response is useful when there is no information about the depth of the abnormality or if deep, mid-line lesions are suspected.

It has been shown that the resolution of a system, as given by the LSF, is dependent on the amount of scattered radiation and, in Chapter 3, that the channel width of a PHA can be set to select photons in the photopeak only, thereby eliminating photons produced by Compton scattering. It is evident that if the channel width is set to too narrow a limit, the number of photons trans-

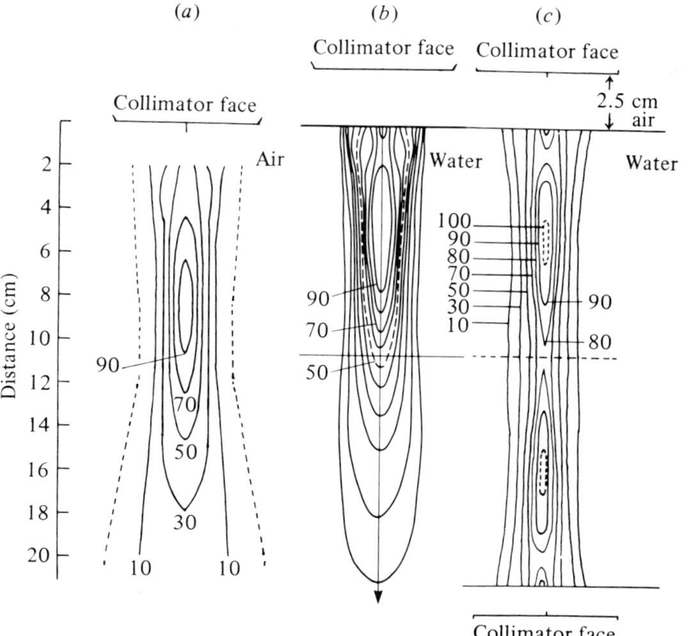

Fig. 7.8. (*a*) and (*b*) Iso-response curves for a single detector with a 10 cm focussed collimator, with a point source of ^{131}I (*a*) in air and (*b*) in water. (*c*) Iso-response curves for two opposing detectors with similar collimators, and the source in water.

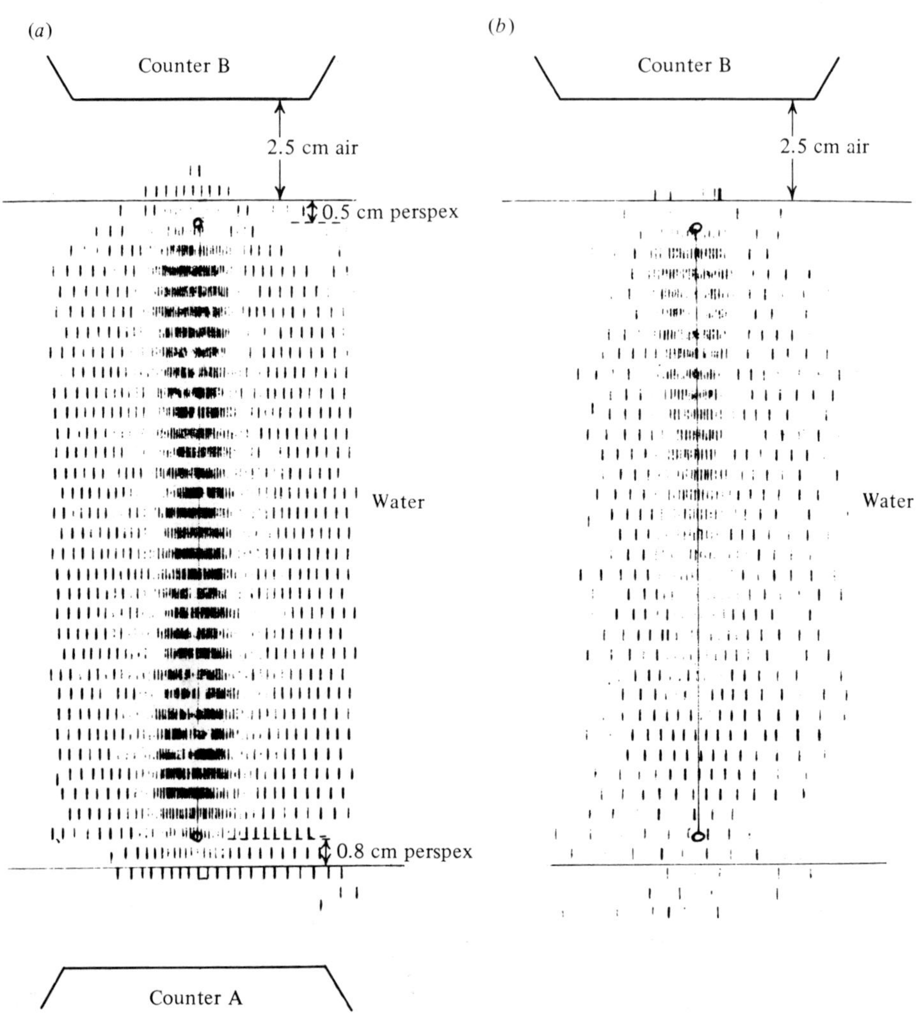

Fig. 7.9. Tapper display of collimator response obtained by carrying out a rectilinear scan on a line source of ^{99m}Tc placed at an angle of 45 degrees to the vertical, in a water tank. The spacing of the tapper marks varies with count-rate, high count-rates being represented by closely spaced marks and low count-rates by wider spaced marks. (*a*) Detectors in parallel; (*b*) single detector.

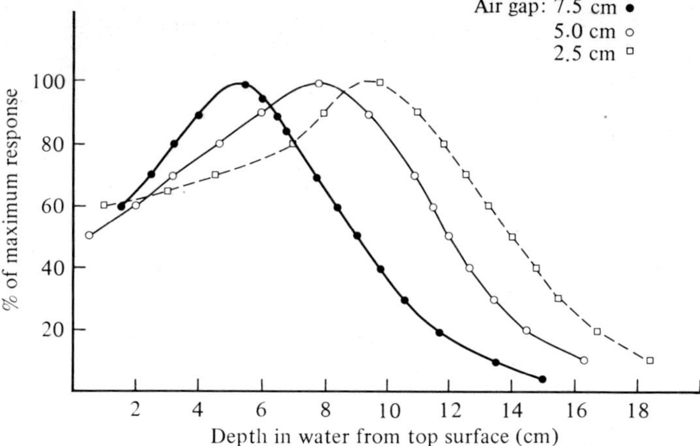

Fig. 7.10. Central-axis depth response curves for a detector with a focussed collimator.

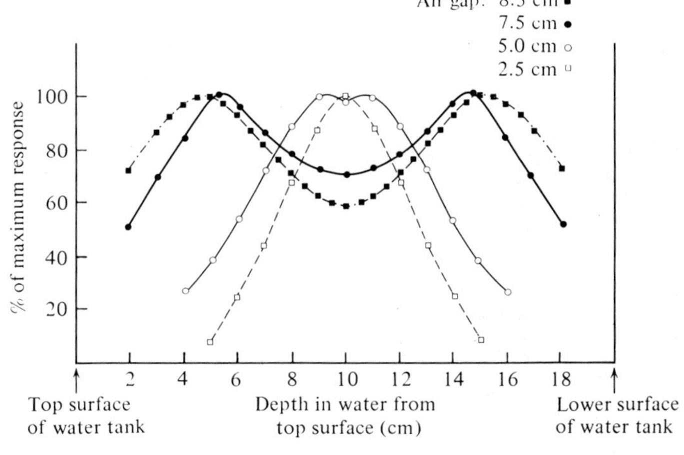

Fig. 7.11. Central-axis depth response curves for two opposing detectors with focussed collimators.

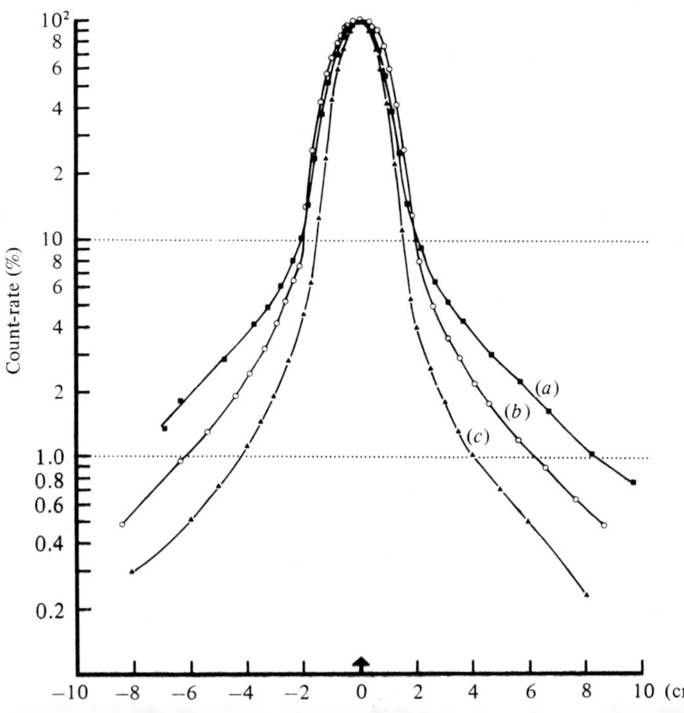

Fig. 7.12. Curves showing the effect of collimation and channel width on resolution. Channel widths: (*a*) 20 V (thin septa); (*b*) 10 V (thin septa); (*c*) 10 V (thick septa).

mitted will be drastically reduced and the sensitivity will be very low. Inevitably a compromise has to be made, and the channel width is usually centred on the photopeak with a width equal to approximately 20–25% of the photopeak energy. For example, for imaging with ^{99m}Tc the channel width should be 0.125–0.160 MeV, with a width of 0.035 MeV, which is 25% of 0.14 MeV.

The effect of collimation and of channel width on resolution is shown in Fig. 7.12. The curves show the variation of response to a line source of ^{99m}Tc across the plane through the focus, perpendicular to the axis. Fig. 7.12(*a*) is the response with a thin septa collimator and a wide channel, (*b*) that with the same collimator and a narrow channel, and (*c*) that with a thick septa collimator of otherwise similar design and a narrow channel. It will be seen that although the difference in FWHM is small, the response curves of the thin septa collimator with the narrow channel show a sharper cut-off of the lower contours (below 10%) than those with the wide channel, and the thick septa collimator improves it even more. This of course is at the expense of reduced sensitivity.

The choice of collimator is, inevitably, a compromise between sensitivity and resolution. The first requirement is that the sensitivity is adequate to carry out the complete investigation in a time which is acceptable to the patient. The depth response of the detector–collimator system must be such that data are collected from the appropriate depth. For example, in the brain, when the lateral views are being scanned with a dual detector system, the whole of each hemisphere will be adequately 'viewed' by the corresponding detector if the depth response is good over 0–7.5 cm water or tissue, with a 2.5 cm air gap. Mid-line structures will be better 'viewed' by summing the data collected from the two detectors. The adrenal glands, which lie fairly superficially, are best viewed with a short-focus collimator focussed at about 6 cm depth.

Information density and display

The photons detected by the NaI crystal may be recorded sequentially as individual pulses, or groups of pulses, by means of a mechanical tapper which produces marks, the spacing of which is proportional to the count-rate (Fig. 7.9). Alternatively, or additionally, the number of pulses detected over a pre-set time, or over a pre-set distance of travel, may be integrated to form an analogue signal, such as a DC voltage, which in turn generates a photographic blackening or a colour code representation of the count-rate.

In the first type of display the pulses which drive the mechanical tapper are nearly always less than the number of pulses at the PHA output. The number is reduced by a constant factor, known as the scaling factor. The choice of the correct scaling factor is important, because it ensures that the mechanical tapper is not overloaded but that the marks are sufficiently close for a good display. In addition it ensures a standard quality of display. It is customary when setting up a scan to centre the detector either over a standard anatomical landmark, or over the area of maximum activity. The speed of scanning is chosen so that a standard information density is obtained for the prescribed area for any particular type of scan, e.g. bone or brain. If the speed of scanning is v cm per minute, the count-rate is C counts per minute and the sampling distance (length of travel over which counts are integrated) is d cm, then the information density (ID), that is the counts collected in one sample element, will be equal to dC/v counts; increasing the speed setting will decrease the ID, and vice versa. In order to obtain reasonable statistics it is advisable to have an ID of the order of 100 counts. Having set the speed to obtain the required ID, the scaling factor can be selected so that the maximum (or any other selected level of) radioactivity records the maximum dot-density, blackening or colour display. There is usually a background subtraction device which permits counts below a pre-set level to be suppressed.

In order to obtain quantitative results it is necessary to record the raw data. There are many forms of data logging equipment; the most common is one which accumulates the pulses from each spatial element of the scan, and records sequentially the number of pulses in each element. The elements may be defined by a predetermined length of scan, e.g. 2, 4 or 5 mm, or by a time interval, e.g. 0.2, 0.4 or 0.5 seconds. The data are often recorded on paper tape; the numbers are represented in code by a series of holes punched in the tape by a paper-tape punch operated by a punch controller. Alternatively, the data may be recorded on magnetic tape or disc. Being in computer-compatible form, the data can then be fed into the computer and processed in a manner similar to that described for gamma cameras (Chapter 9).

Procedure

To summarise the operation of a rectilinear scanner:

(1) Set the detector operating conditions for the radionuclide being used.
(2) Choose the correct collimator and air gap.
(3) Set up the equipment over the patient, centring either over a standard position or over the highest activity, according to standard practice.
 3.1. Choose the speed to get a good ID, consistent with an acceptable overall scanning time.
 3.2. Select scaling factor for correct display.
 3.3. Set the background subtract.
(4) Carry out the scan.
(5) Insert anatomical landmarks as required.
(6) Take an X-ray if required.

Quality control
When a rectilinear scanner is installed, measurements should be made of stability, sensitivity and spatial and energy resolution, and results checked against the manufacturer's specification. The mechanical movement, the speed and spacing should be checked, as should also the accuracy with which the movement of the display system follows that of the detector system. The relationship between the count-rate and the colour, or photographic density range, should be investigated to ensure it follows the required law, e.g. linear or logarithmic.

Subsequently, weekly measurements should be made of the photopeak position of, for example, ^{99m}Tc, and of sensitivity using a long-term standard. Records should be kept, and trends or large fluctuations investigated. The quality of the display should be critically examined at regular intervals, and the mechanical movement carefully inspected.

New developments
Since the introduction of technetium-labelled phosphate compounds for bone imaging, there has in most centres been a great increase in the work-load. It is becoming a widely accepted policy that radionuclide imaging should precede radiological skeletal surveys. There is therefore a need for equipment to carry out rapid bone imaging studies.

Such a piece of equipment was first proposed by Anger and developed commercially by Picker in 1968, and was known as the Dynapix (Verdon & Allen, 1969, p. 177). The essential feature was the use of a rectangular detector of overall size 25 cm by

Fig. 7.14. Isoresponse curves for each crystal of the Cleon Scanner. (Reproduced by permission of Internuclear Ltd.)

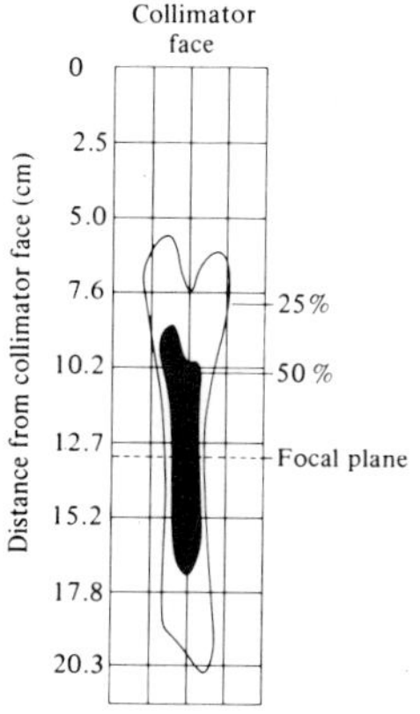

2.5 cm, consisting of 10 NaI crystals each of size 2.5 cm square, arranged in the form of a strip. A single longitudinal sweep recorded 10 scan lines (with 2.5 cm spacing) simultaneously, and then by causing the detector to step transversely and repeat the longitudinal sweep, scan lines between the initial 10 were obtained.

More recently the Cleon Scanner (Fig. 7.13) was produced by the Cleon Corporation, following the design of Smith & Katchie (1969). It carries the option of a single or dual detector system, with one detector above and one below the moving couch. Each detector head contains an array of 10 NaI crystals in a configuration 60 cm by 11.5 cm, and 10 scan lines, at 6.1 cm spacing, are recorded simultaneously. Each crystal has its own focussed collimater; the characteristics of the long-focus collimator are shown in Fig. 7.14, which shows a FWHM of 9 mm at 13.2 cm in air. The length of the sampling element may be set to 1.9, 3.8 or 7.6 mm; with a FWHM of 9 mm the optimum size is probable 3.8 mm, but 7.6 mm is normally used in the interest of speed. The detectors make one longitudinal sweep. At each sampling element the detector heads scan transversely by one crystal's width, thereby scanning the whole width; the detectors then advance longitudinally by one element and the procedure is repeated. All the data are collected on magnetic disc and can be read back for 'minified' display on a TV monitor, or for permanent photographic display.

The system is built so that the highest count-rate, or any other selected count-rate, is automatically displayed at maximum

Fig. 7.13. A multi-crystal rectilinear scanner. (Reproduced by permission of Internuclear Ltd.)

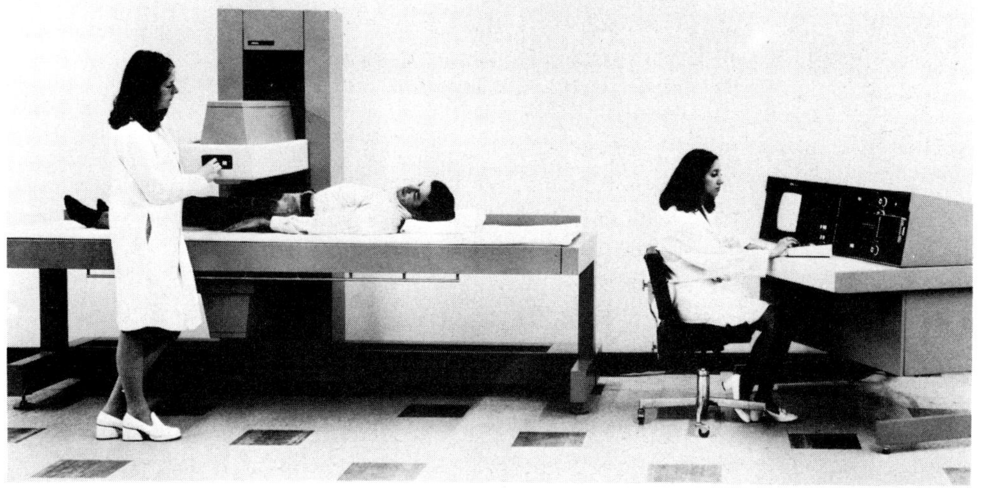

blackening, and any required degree of background cut-off may be used. The great advantage of this system, apart from that of speed, is that it obviates the necessity of searching for the region of highest activity when setting up; also the facility of retrospective variable background cut-off enables bone scans with EHDP or MDP to be carried out at about 1 hour after injection instead of 3 or 4 hours (Ell *et al.*, 1977). A skeletal survey carried out on this machine at half an hour after injection is shown in Fig. 7.15(*a*), and one at the usual 3 hours in (*b*).

Gamma cameras

A gamma camera has a large detector which looks at the radiation from the whole of the field of view simultaneously. The detector may be a single large NaI crystal as in the Anger camera or a matrix of small crystals as in the Autofluoroscope. Both of these look at the whole depth of tissue in the field of view, and produce a two-dimensional image of a three-dimensional object. As with the rectilinear scanner, section imaging can be achieved with specialised equipment.

Fig. 7.15. Image of skeleton obtained using the Cleon Scanner. (*a*) Scan carried out at half an hour after injection (with subtraction); (*b*) scan carried out at 3 hours after injection (raw data). (Scintigram kindly provided by Dr P. Ell, Middlesex Hospital.)

(*a*) (*b*)

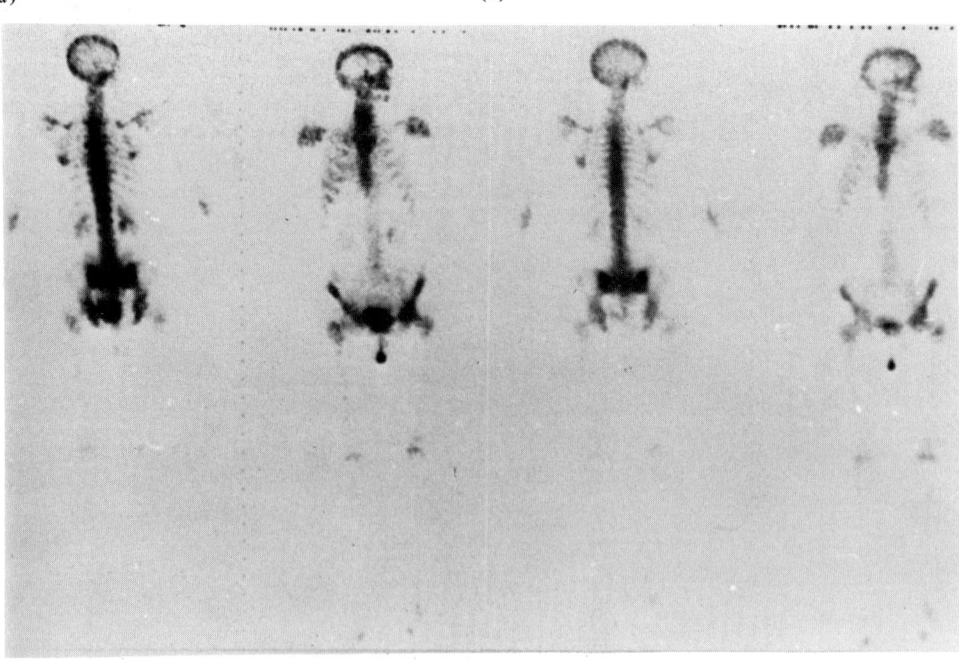

Post. Ant. Post. Ant.

Single-crystal cameras

A photograph of a modern gamma camera is shown in Fig. 7.16(a), together with a diagram in Fig. 7.16(b). It consists essentially of a

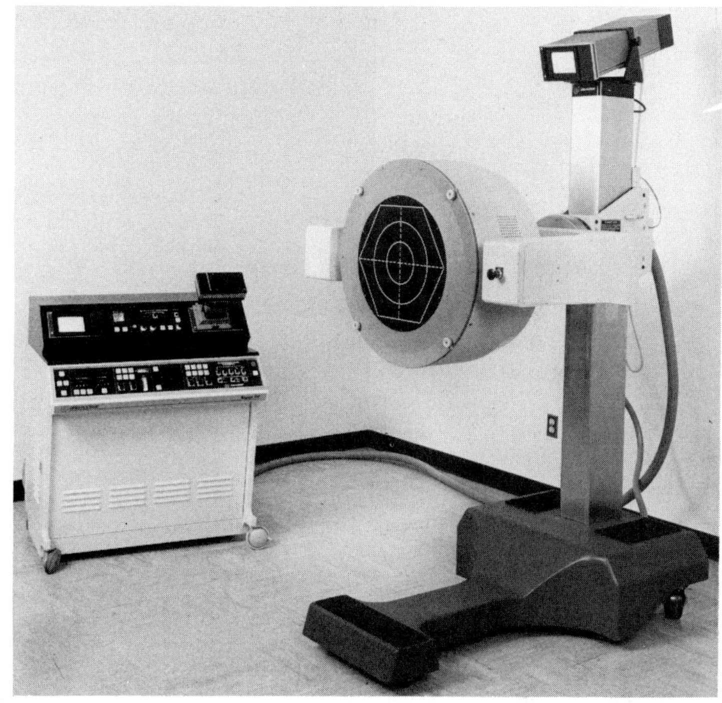

(a)

Fig. 7.16. (a) A modern gamma camera. (Photograph kindly provided by Ohio Nuclear Ltd.) (b) Diagram of gamma camera. (Reproduced from G. Hine (ed.) (1967), *Instrumentation in Nuclear Medicine*, vol. 1, by kind permission of the publishers Academic Press.)

(b)

X^+
X^-
Y^+
Y^-
Output signals
Capacitor network
Lead shield
Hexagonal array of 19 PM tubes
Light deflector
Optical light-guide
NaI crystal
Glass window of crystal housing
Multichannel collimator

large NaI crystal viewed by an array of photomultiplier (PM) tubes. A computing circuit, used to analyse the signals from the PM tubes, senses the position of scintillations in the crystal and provides three output pulses for each scintillation event; the X and Y pulses give the coordinates and the Z pulse is proportional to the brightness of the scintillation. These output pulses are transmitted to an oscilloscope which reproduces the scintillations as point flashes of light at the correct locations. In this way a picture is built up on the oscilloscope of the radiation source being imaged. A permanent record can be achieved by photographing the image on the oscilloscope. The position of each scintillation in the crystal is accurately determined by analysis of the proportional division of light among the PM tubes, and with a modern 37-PM tube camera it is possible to assign a location within a matrix of 256 by 256 elements, which with a field of view of 10 inch (25 cm) diameter corresponds to 1 mm^2 elements.

The factors which need to be taken into account when using a gamma camera will now be considered.

Field uniformity. The NaI scintillation crystal operates in the same way as described in Chapter 3, and the associated equipment is similar. However, since there are many PM tubes each has to have its own high-voltage (HV) supply, and the gain of each has to be adjusted to produce a uniform field of view, a process referred to as tuning. There is usually a common HV supply, together with a small independent potentiometer control for each PM tube. Tuning, with some gamma cameras, is done by the manufacturers, but with other modern cameras is easily done by using a Z-pulse monitor oscilloscope to bring the photopeak of, for example, a ^{99m}Tc source, within the pre-set window for each PM tube.

With the gamma camera there is an inherent problem of uniformity which does not arise with the rectilinear scanner, because in the latter the whole field is viewed sequentially by the same detector. The cause of non-uniformity may be spatial variations in sensitivity or spatial distortions. Any observed non-uniformity is due to a combination of the above two causes. The most common method of assessing field uniformity, and the one specified in the IEC draft document 62C, is that of imaging a flood field phantom. The measurement is carried out using a uniform source, usually of ^{99m}Tc, of dimensions larger than the field of view. It is performed using an appropriate parallel-hole collimator, and the

(a)

Fig. 7.17. Polaroid pictures of a flood field image: (a) Uniform image; (b) non-uniform image due to operation off the photopeak. (c) grossly non-uniform image due to failure of one PM tube.

(b)

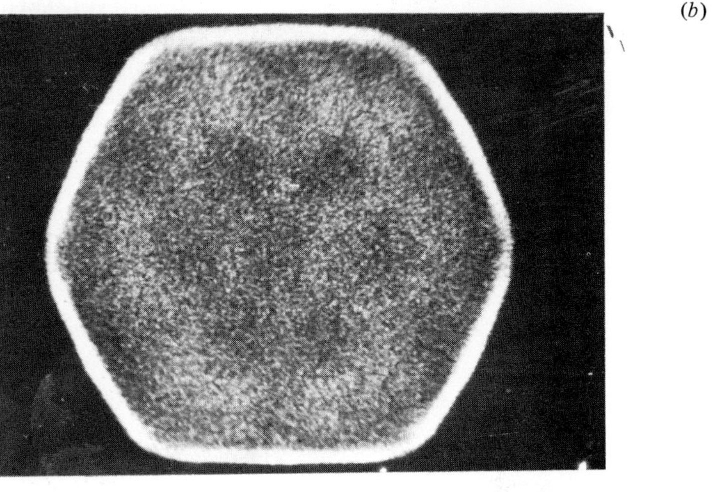

(c)

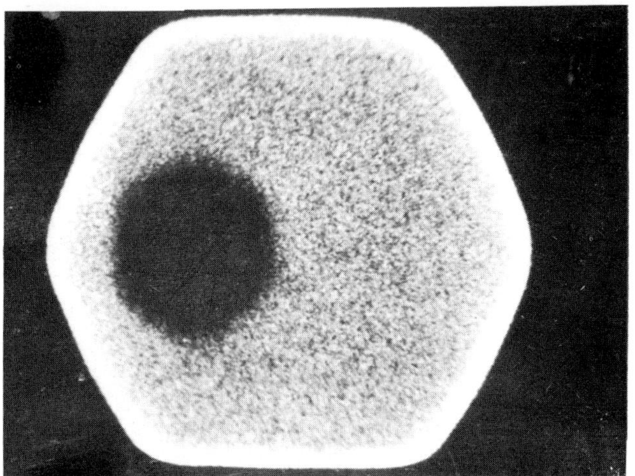

source is placed as close as possible to the collimator surface. An image is obtained by collecting 500 000 counts for the usual photographic display. The IEC document requires that data (more than 10 000 counts) are collected for each small area of the field, and that the mean and standard deviation of these counts is calculated. For purposes of routine imaging, to be interpreted by visual inspection, the photographic display of the flood field source is obviously the critical one, since any non-uniformity in this would be present in any image and may lead to mis-diagnosis. In Fig. 7.17, (*a*) shows a uniform flood field image, (*b*) shows a non-uniform flood field image such as is obtained when the camera is not operated on the photopeak, and (*c*) shows a gross non-uniformity obtained when one PM tube was not operating.

If flood field data are collected as a matrix of numbers, a correction can be applied to images that are data-processed (Chapter 9), and this has been common practice. However, Todd-Pokropek (Todd-Pokropek *et al.*, 1977) has pointed out that because these numbers include non-uniformity defects due to variations in both sensitivity and spatial distortion if present, this correction is not necessarily valid for quantitation. Variations in sensitivity only, may be quantitated by measurements on a collimated point source placed at each small area of the field in turn, and corrections based on these should be used for quantitative work. However, these measurements are laborious, and not suitable for routine work. Some modern cameras use microprocessor techniques to apply corrections.

Collimation, sensitivity and resolution. As with the rectilinear scanner, operating conditions with regard to channel width and collimation are a compromise between sensitivity and resolution. The optimum channel base-line for ^{99m}Tc has been shown to be 0.125–0.127 MeV when the energy resolution is 15.9% (Atkins *et al.*, 1977); the upper limit is not so critical, and is usually set to 0.160 MeV.

The sensitivity of a gamma camera as specified in the IEC document is measured in the same way as for a rectilinear scanner but with the plane source at 10 cm from the collimator face. The plane sensitivity will be independent of distance in air, but is depth-dependent in water because of absorption and scatter.

The resolution of a gamma camera may also be defined in the same way as for a rectilinear scanner, that is, as the FWHM of a line spread function (LSF). It should be appreciated, however, that the gamma camera has a power of resolution even without collimation. This is known as the intrinsic resolution and it represents the best possible LSF which the system could achieve if it had perfect collimation. The degradation shown in the intrinsic LSF is due to the image converter and is caused by loss of positional resolution in the NaI crystal because of Compton scattering, statistical uncertainty due to low number of photons, and imperfections in the light guide.

A plane source of radioactivity placed in contact with the detector face will produce an image, the quality of which will be dependent on the intrinsic resolution. With a solid source, collimation is required to select the γ-rays that proceed from it in a direction perpendicular to the crystal face, in order that the location of an ionising event in the crystal may correspond, within the overall resolution of the system, to the origin of the γ-ray producing it. The collimators, therefore, are cylindrical blocks of lead in which are drilled multiple, small, usually parallel, holes (Fig. 7.16*b*). Sometimes a diverging-hole collimator may be used to provide a larger field of view, or a converging-hole collimator to give some magnification; both give poorer resolution than a parallel-hole collimator with the same sized holes and septa at the crystal face. Occasionally a pin-hole collimator may be used for thin, superficial sources, as for example the lacrymal ducts.

With collimation, the overall resolution is given by:

$$R_o^2 = R_c^2 + R_i^2$$

where R_o = overall resolution
R_c = collimator resolution
R_i = intrinsic resolution

and

$$R_c = \frac{d}{L}(Z + L + t) \text{ for a parallel-hole collimator}$$

where d = hole diameter
L = length of collimator
t = septal thickness
Z = distance from collimator face

Test conditions for measuring both intrinsic and overall LSF are specified in the IEC document. The measurement involves the use of either data logging and computer facilities, a multi-channel analyser, or a microdensitometer to produce the curve of count-rate versus distance from the central axis of the line source.

Fig. 7.18 shows the overall LSF for a gamma camera with a high-resolution collimator, with a ^{99m}Tc line source at a depth of 2 cm in water.

The resolution of gamma cameras is often assessed subjectively, using test patterns of different types. The most commonly used is the Anger phantom, which has hexagonal arrays of holes of different sizes in a lead disc. Fig. 7.19 shows the result obtained with an Ohio Nuclear camera and the test phantom in contact with the face of the detector to demonstrate intrinsic resolution; it shows that the smallest hole, of diameter 2 mm, with spacing of 8 mm, is clearly seen at count-rates of 6.8×10^3 counts per second but the image deteriorates when the count-rate is increased to 37.2×10^3 counts per second (see next section).

Haematocrit tubes, of internal diameter 1 mm, make useful line sources when filled with radioactive solutions, and results with these sources placed parallel to each other at different spacings may be obtained at different depths in water (Fig. 7.20). The degradation of the image with increased depth is evident.

Fig. 7.18. Line spread function for a gamma camera. (The photograph opposite shows the original print-out.)

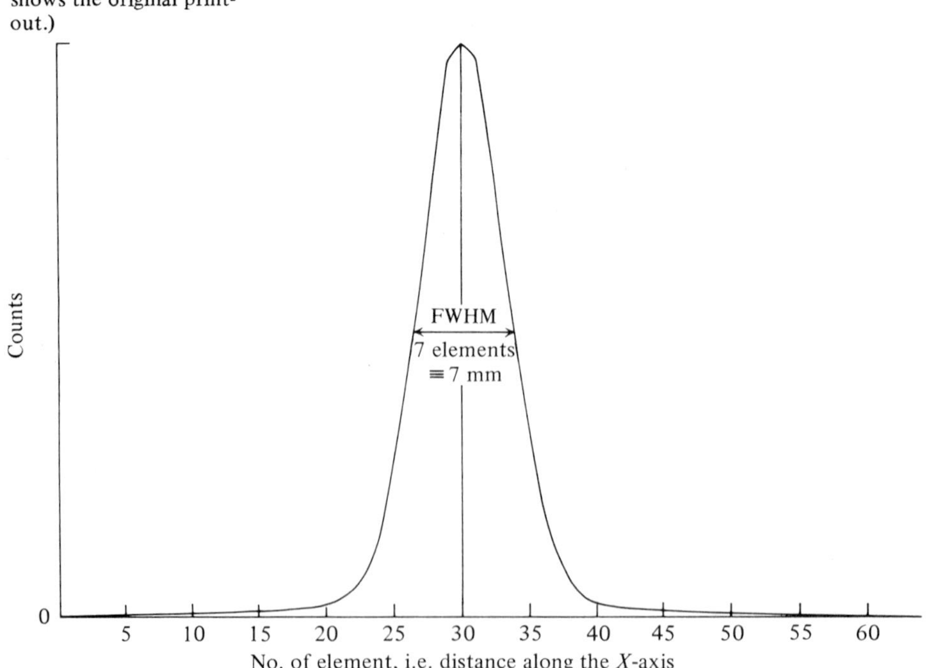

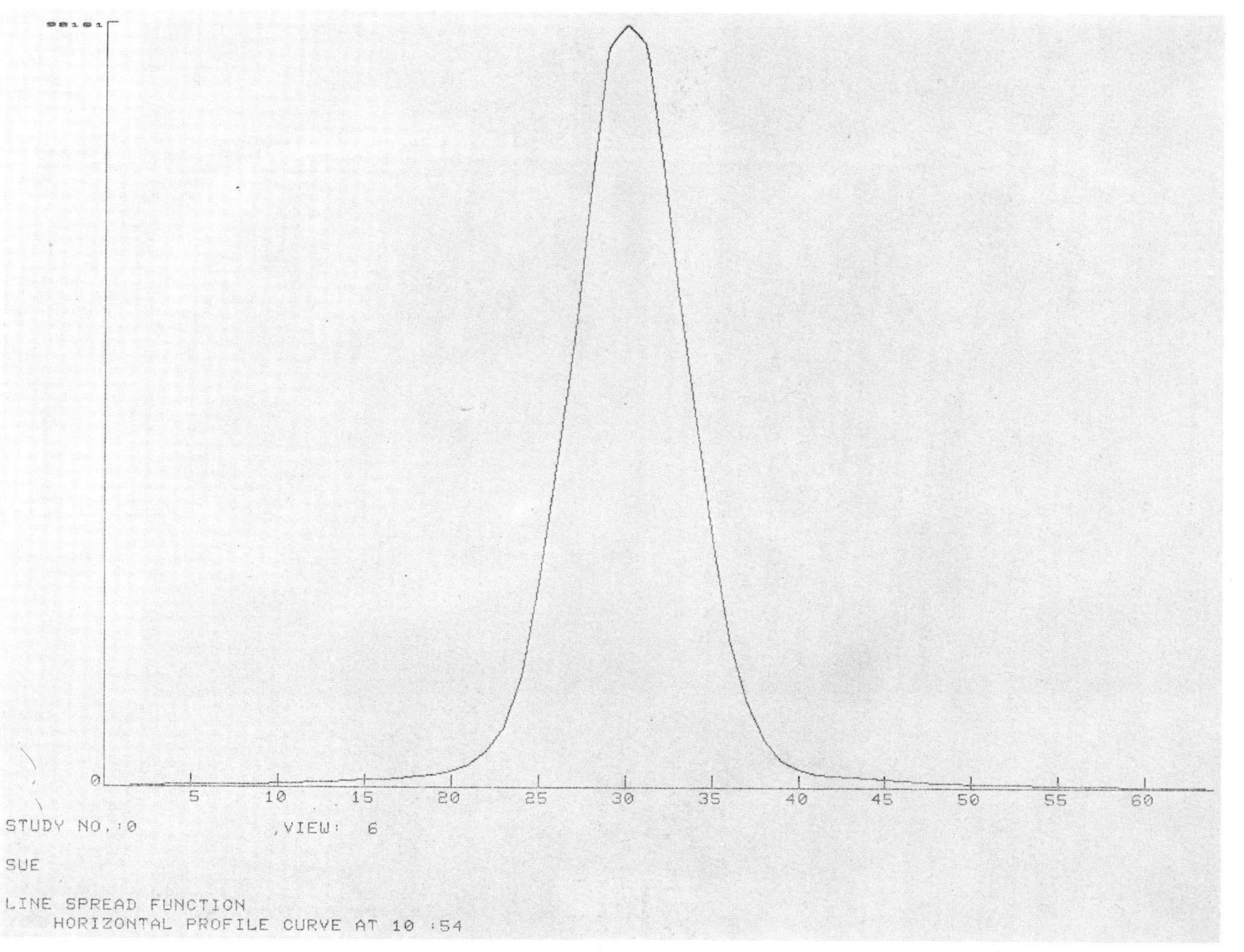
98181
0
5
10
15
20
25
30
35
40
45
50
55
60
STUDY NO.:0 ,VIEW: 6
SUE
LINE SPREAD FUNCTION
HORIZONTAL PROFILE CURVE AT 10 :54

Fig. 7.19. Polaroid pictures of the image of an Anger phantom. (*a*) Obtained using a count-rate of 6.8×10^3 counts per second; (*b*) obtained using a count-rate of 37.2×10^3 counts per second, and demonstrating deterioration of the image.

(*a*)

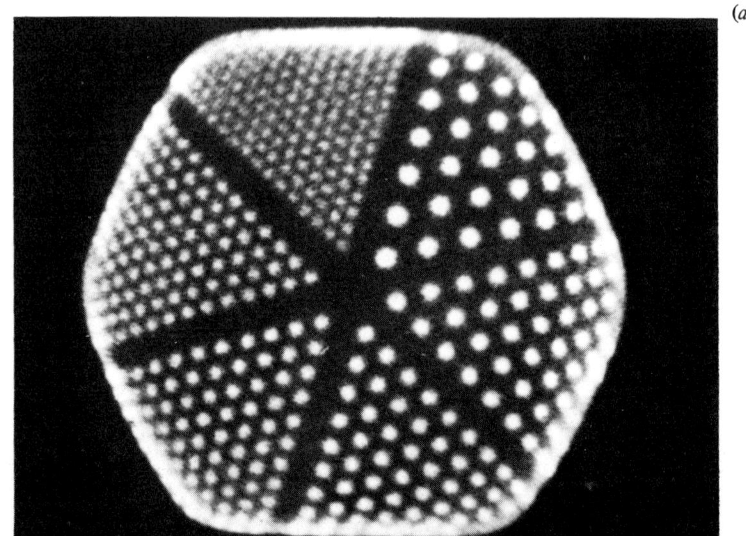

(*b*)

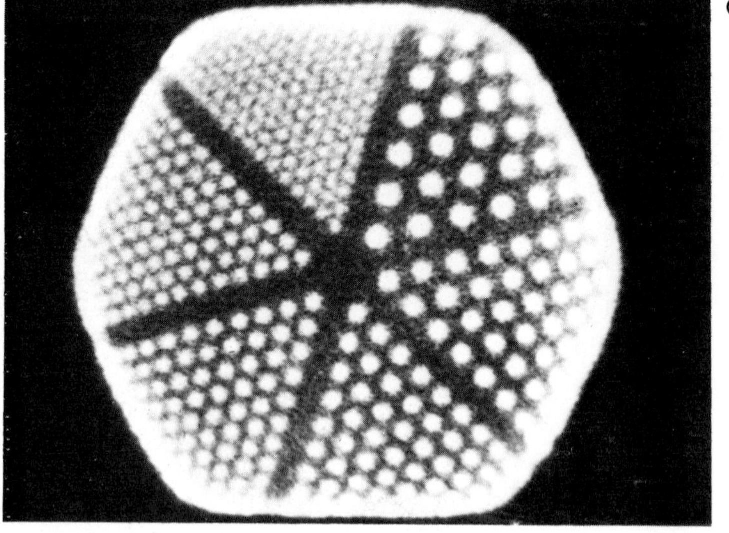

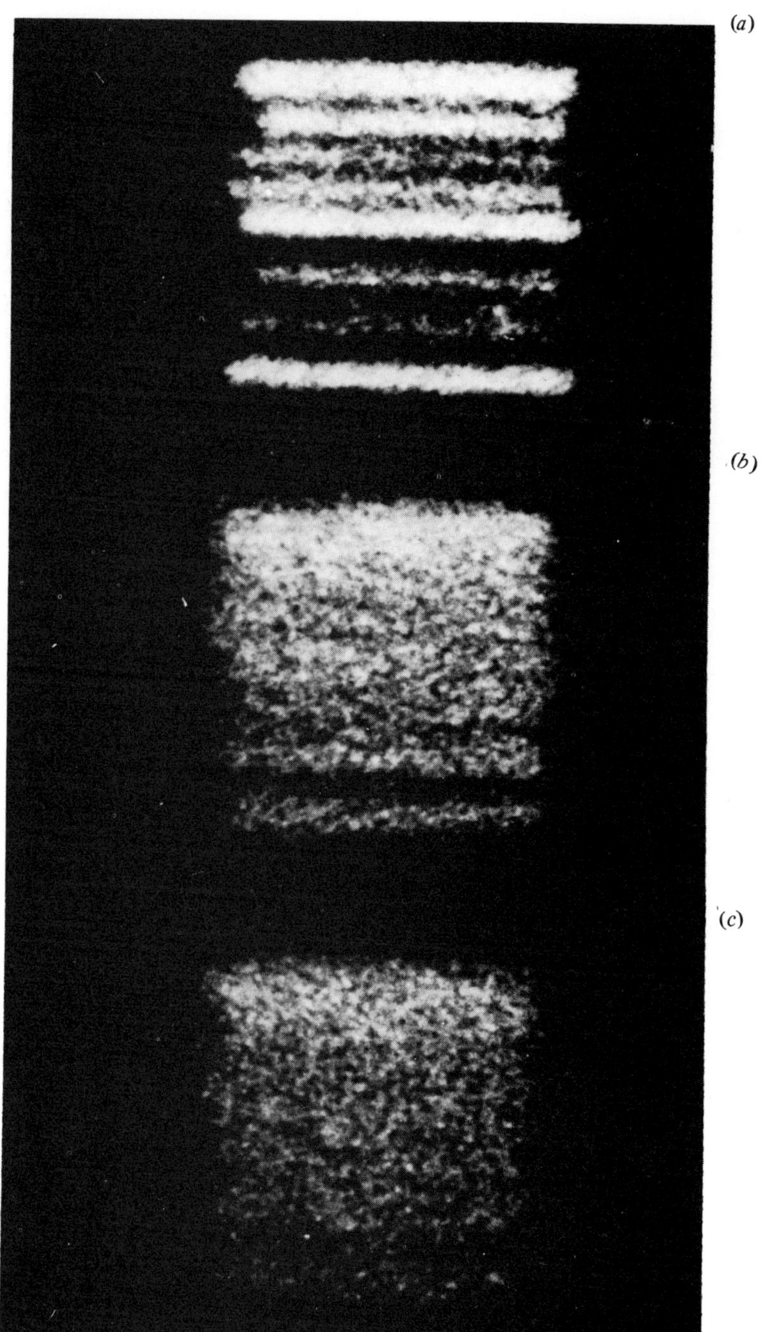

Fig. 7.20. Polaroid pictures of images of spaced line sources of ^{99m}Tc. (*a*) In contact with the collimator face; (*b*) and (*c*) at depths of 4.8 cm and 9.4 cm, in a scattering medium.

Loss of counts and resolution at high count-rates. The problems encountered at high count-rates as a result of counting losses and pile-up were referred to in Chapter 4. It was shown that there are two types of dead-time: paralysable and non-paralysable. A gamma camera is considered to be a system with a paralysable component followed by a non-paralysable component. Sorensen (1976) has investigated three methods of dead-time correction. The first of these is an analytical method, as described in Chapter 4, involving measurement of camera dead-time and the use of mathematical expressions to obtain correction factors for observed count-rates under various experimental conditions; this method proved to be inaccurate. The second method uses a shielded, small-volume marker source placed on the periphery of the detector, counts from this source being monitored during the study; changes in the count-rate are presumed to reflect changes in dead-time losses over the entire detector. The third method is based on the assumption that the loss of counts is proportional to the number of pile-up events recorded in a channel above the photopeak. Using ^{99m}Tc sources of increasing strength, the author obtained the ratio of the counts in a 35% window centred at 220 KeV, to the counts in the 140 KeV photopeak window, and plotted this ratio against the ratio of true to observed counts. A straight line resulted, showing that the dead-time correction can be made by this method. It was concluded that this is the best method of correcting for dead-time, but the author pointed out that it may not be applicable with some new cameras which have improved pile-up rejection circuits.

There is one important difference between cameras and counters which causes another problem, namely that the camera must assign position coordinates (addresses) to the scintillations. When, at high count-rates, the pile-up effect occurs and scintillations sum up randomly, new false addresses are generated which in clinical images cannot be distinguished from true addresses. This effect has been investigated by Lange (Lange *et al.*, 1977). Using three point sources of ^{99m}Tc positioned at the apices of a triangle, and setting the PHA of the camera to 280 KeV, he showed that false images were produced at the apices of the triangle due to pile-up of two 140 KeV photoevents, and between the apices due to pile-up of Compton scattering events. It follows that true addresses will be lost from the 140 KeV photopeak window, and false addresses produced due to pile-up of lower energy Compton scattering events. This effect could cause serious problems with sources of strength greater than 10–20 mCi, and there is at present no known method for measuring or calculating regional correction factors; but the problem may be solved by the use of built-in pile-up rejection circuits.

Spatial linearity. Another inherent problem with the gamma camera that does not arise with the rectilinear scanner is that of spatial distortion. Linearity is dependent on the accurate assignment of the *X* and *Y* coordinates. The use of light guides in camera design tends to give rise to some spatial distortion, although improving resolution. Fig. 7.21 shows an image of a series of line sources, and demonstrates that barrel distortion is present at the periphery of the field of view.

Display. As described above, the image is displayed on an oscilloscope, and a permanent record may be obtained by photographing this image on Polaroid or transparent film.

Polaroid film has the advantage of being immediately available for inspection, but the disadvantages of high contrast, coarseness of grain, and considerable variation in photographic quality, e.g. speed and contrast, from batch to batch. Transparent film has the disadvantages of requiring processing, and the delay while this is done, but the improvement in quality makes it very worthwhile. Most gamma cameras produce, for routine purposes a minified image of size 100 mm by 100 mm, others have facilities for a 70 mm roll film for rapid sequential imaging, and some produce a life-size photographic record. The intensity of blackening will depend on the rate at which light flashes are produced on the oscilloscope, the intensity of the light flashes, and the time of exposure, and also on the camera aperture and characteristics of the film. The intensity of the light flashes is controlled by the intensity setting of the scope, and this is usually fixed for any particular investigation, as are also the camera stop and the type of film. For static studies it is usual to collect a pre-set number of counts; it is evident that the quality of the image will depend on the distribution of the radioactivity and that in order to obtain a consistent quality it is necessary to use a standard configuration. For example, in static brain imaging a total count of 300 000 is used; but the activity in the facial muscles is appreciably higher than that in the brain, and therefore if a large area of the face is included the number of counts arising from the brain will be significantly less than 300 000 and the image of the brain will be

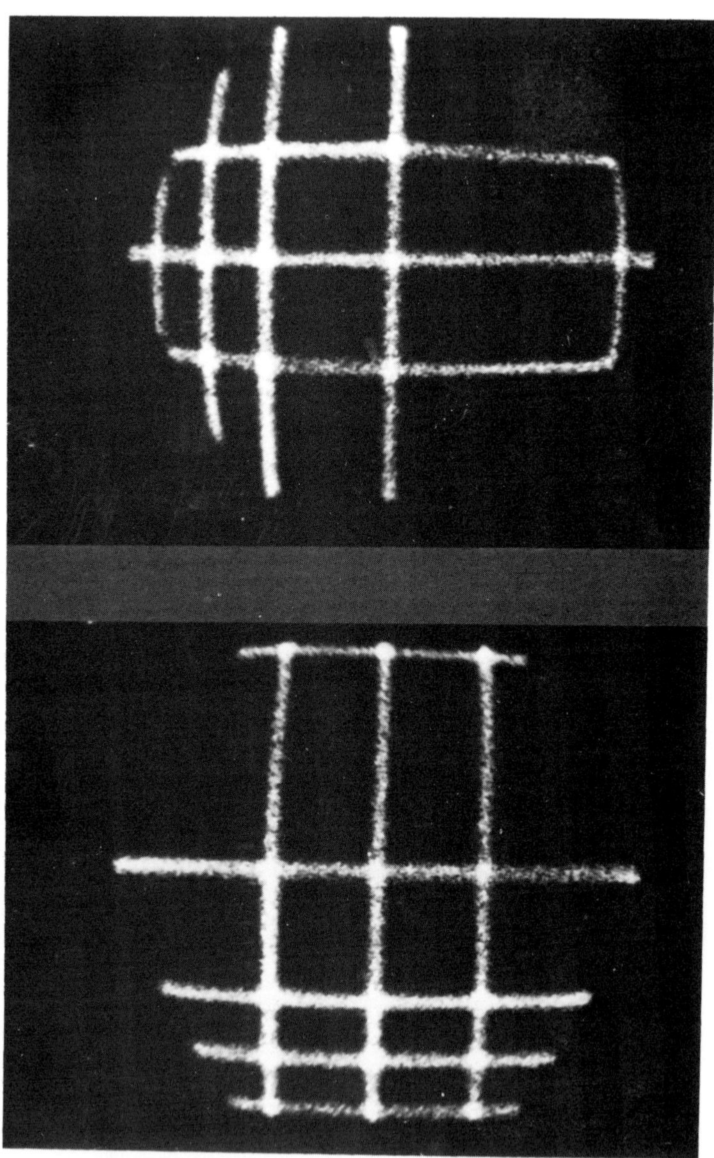

Fig. 7.21. Polaroid pictures of the image of a phantom made up from straight-line sources, showing some barrel distortion at the periphery.

under-exposed. This applies particularly in lateral views. In order to get comparable views on a patient it is sometimes helpful to time the first exposure of 300 000 counts and expose the other views for that same time.

More sophisticated forms of display are described in Chapter 9.

Data collection and data processing. Most gamma cameras have data collection and data processing facilities. These will be discussed in Chapter 9.

Procedure. To summarise the operation of a gamma camera:

(1) Set the detector operating conditions for the radionuclide being used.

(2) Choose the correct collimator.

(3) Set the intensity factor for the oscilloscope.

(4) Check that the correct camera back is in position and loaded. Set the camera aperture to the correct value.

(5) Set the gamma camera to record counts for pre-set time or pre-set counts.

(6) Set the computer, if it is being used, to acquire the data in the required mode; there will normally be a protocol for each routine investigation and then it is only necessary to call the appropriate protocol.

(7) Position the camera and patient, watching the image which builds up on the persistence oscilloscope to ensure that the projection is accurate, and also that the region under investigation is correctly sited within the field of view.

(8) Expose the photographic film by opening the shutter for the required time; there may or may not be automatic exposure.

Quality control. When a gamma camera is installed measurements should be made of stability, field uniformity, plane sensitivity, LSF, spatial linearity and count-rate capability. Results should be compared with the manufacturer's specifications.

Subsequently weekly checks should be made of the tuning of the PM tubes, and any continuous trend, or large variations, should be noted and investigated. A photograph of a flood field source should be taken daily and inspected for field uniformity before the camera is put into clinical use. Regular checks of sensitivity should also be made.

The Hospital Physicists' Association and the US Department

Fig. 7.22. A multi-crystal camera. (Photograph kindly provided by Baird-Atomic Inc.)

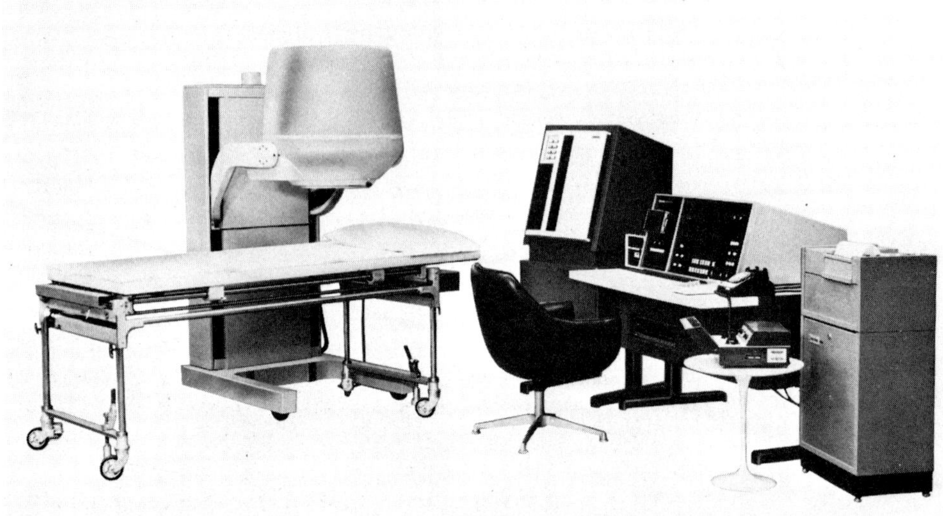

Fig. 7.23. Array of 21 × 14 NaI crystals in multi-crystal camera. (Photograph kindly provided by Baird-Atomic Inc.)

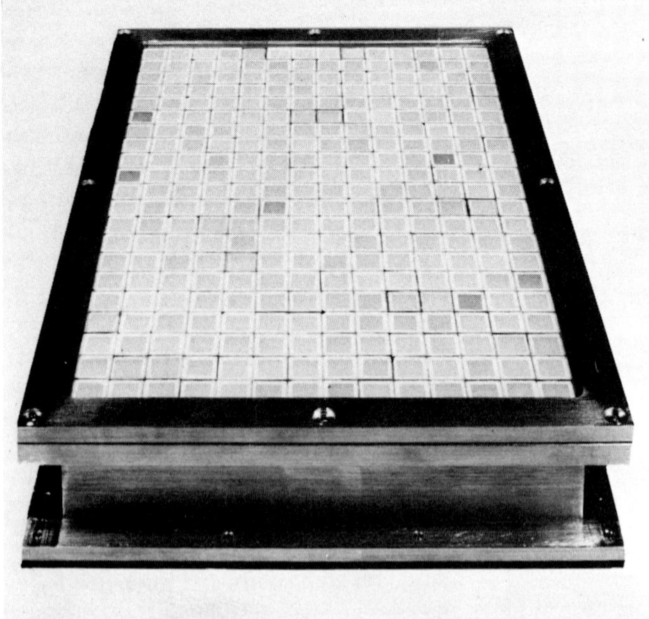

of Health, Education and Welfare both publish useful documents that give guidance on quality control of gamma cameras (HPA, 1977; USDHEW, 1977).

Multi-crystal cameras

The building of a camera with an array of small crystals was conceived and executed by Bender (Bender & Blau, 1963) and he called it an Autofluoroscope. Such a device was first built commercially in 1970 by Baird-Atomic, who remain the sole manufacturers of this type of camera. The following refers to their System Seventy-Seven, a photograph of which is shown in Fig. 7.22. Fig. 7.23 shows the array of 294 crystals, each with a square cross-section of side $\frac{5}{16}$ inch (7.9 mm) and of depth 1.5 inches (38 mm). The 294 crystals are optically coupled to 35 PM tubes by means of a light-pipe assembly (Fig. 7.24). Each crystal has two light pipes so placed that one-half of the light from each scintillation event is guided down each pipe, to the appropriate two PM tubes, and in this way each crystal is uniquely 'addressed'. It should be noted that, in contrast to the Anger camera, the system has virtually no intrinsic resolution, this being in fact the

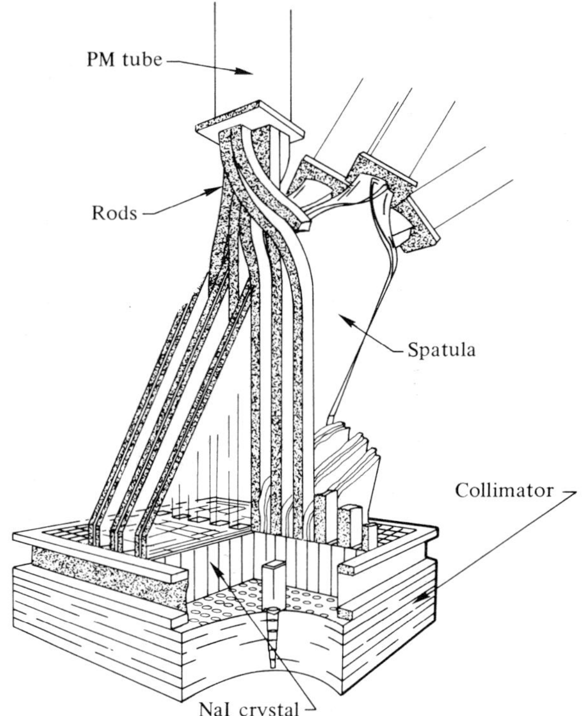

Fig. 7.24. Light-pipe assembly for multi-crystal camera. (Photograph kindly provided by Baird-Atomic Inc.)

centre-to-centre distance between the crystals, which is $\frac{7}{16}$ inch (11.1 mm). The collimator system almost completely defines the imaging properties. Parallel-multi-hole collimators limit the field of view of each crystal detector, with respect to the source of radioactivity; there is a single tapered hole for each crystal. In principle, spatial resolution is limited only by the collimator and sample cell size, if there is no intrinsic component of resolution. The optimum cell size that should be used is a function of FWHM and the count-rate. In order to reduce the sample cell size, which in normal mode is the same as the crystal spacing, the crystal array may be moved, with respect to the source, 16 times with increments equal to one-quarter of the centre-to-centre spacing. The movement is in practice achieved by moving the bed on which the patient is lying. In this way, each detector collects data from 16 sampling points spaced at one-quarter of the crystal-to-crystal distance. It is evident that the handling of the accumulated data requires computer processing, and the system incorporates a buffer memory to store events during the accumulation mode, and a programmable computer interfaced to a rotating memory.

This system may be used for static and dynamic studies. It

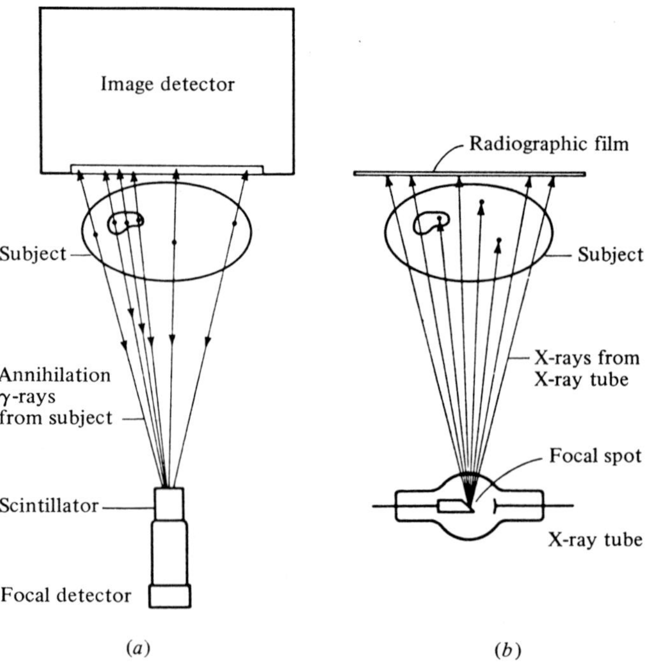

Fig. 7.25. (*a*) Schematic diagram of a simple positron camera. (*b*) Diagram showing analogy with an X-ray tube. (Reproduced from G. Hine (ed.) (1967), *Instrumentation in Nuclear Medicine*, vol. 1, by kind permission of the publishers Academic Press.)

should be appreciated that the high spatial resolution attained by the use of the movable bed is only obtainable for static studies. For dynamic studies spatial resolution is in theory limited by the sampling area but in practice higher spatial resolution is achieved by temporal resolution. These studies will be discussed in Chapter 9.

Positron cameras

It will be recalled that when a positron comes to rest in matter, it combines with an electron and produces two 0.51 MeV annihilation γ-rays which travel in opposite directions from their point of origin. This property allows images to be formed with two detectors on opposite sides of the patient, using coincidence circuitry to record only those positrons from which a γ-ray is received in both detectors. This of course means that the combined detectors have position-sensing capabilities. The simplest form of positron camera is shown in Fig. 7.25(*a*). On one side, placed close to the patient, is a straightforward gamma camera as described above but with no collimator, and on the other an ordinary scintillation counter with a large thick crystal located some distance away. This crystal is called a focal detector because one γ-ray of each annihilation pair must reach it in order that the other γ-ray of the pair may be recorded as a coincidence in the gamma camera, and therefore the second γ-ray must proceed in a straight line from the focal detector. The analogy with the focal spot of an X-ray tube is demonstrated in Fig. 7.25(*b*). By using two gamma cameras or a more complex focal detector it is possible to get a focussing effect. This will be considered in more detail in the following section on tomography.

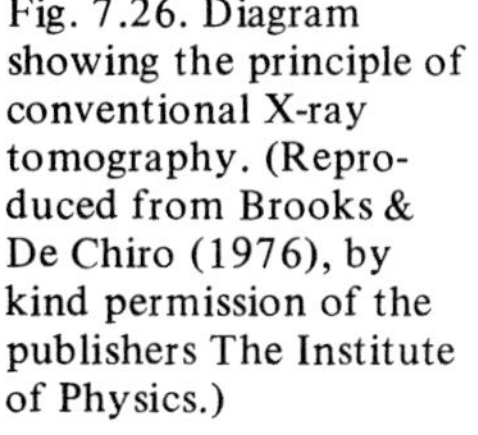

Fig. 7.26. Diagram showing the principle of conventional X-ray tomography. (Reproduced from Brooks & De Chiro (1976), by kind permission of the publishers The Institute of Physics.)

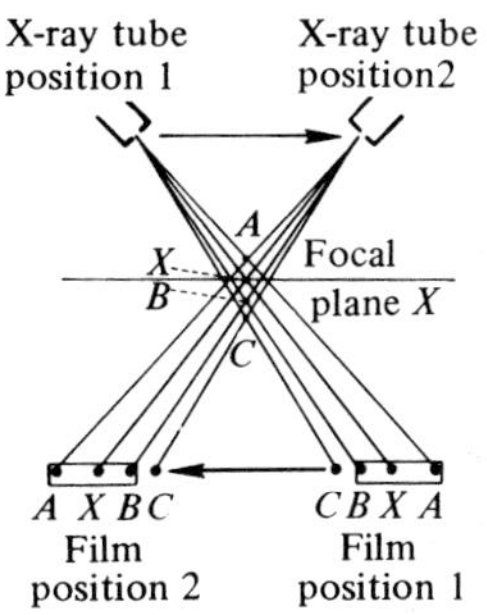

Tomography

Tomography is, as its name implies, the displaying of a slice or section. X-ray transmission focal-plane tomography has been used in conventional radiography since about 1930, and the principle is demonstrated in Fig. 7.26. By moving the X-ray tube and the film relative to each other during exposure, objects in planes other than the plane of interest are blurred out, whereas objects in the plane of interest are sharply defined. In radionuclide imaging, a partial focal-plane tomographic effect can be achieved by using a short-focus collimator focussed at the plane of interest; a high response is obtained from objects in that plane relative to those in other planes (Fig. 7.8*b*).

More sophisticated focal-plane tomography was first suggested by Kuhl & Edwards (1963) and Anger (1969). The principle of Anger's longitudinal tomographic system is shown in Fig. 7.27. It utilises a conventional gamma camera with a conventional focussed collimator, and this detector system scans across the object. Fig. 7.27 shows the area of the crystal which is irradiated by a point source of radioactivity placed at each of the 25 locations. By using a suitable optical readout (Anger, 1968) or computer program (Myers, Keyes & Mallard, 1973) the image may be moved in synchronism with the detector so that for one particular plane the image is always in focus. By using five different factors to relate the detector movement and the image movement, it is possible to build up images of five different planes simultaneously. Fig. 7.28 shows in (*a*) three radioactive sources on planes *A*, *C* and *E*, in (*b*) the motion of the detector during scan as seen from above,

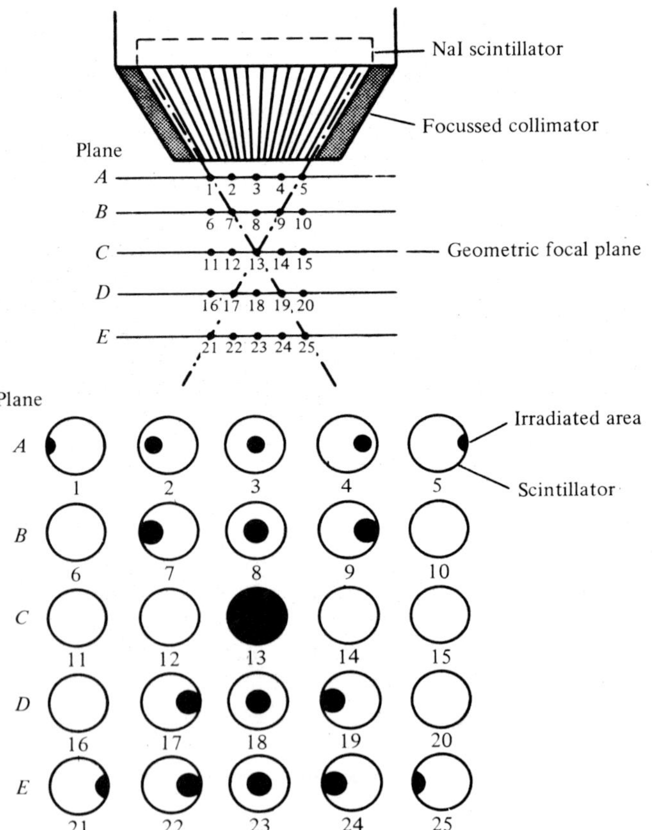

Fig. 7.27. Diagram showing the principle of longitudinal tomography. (Reproduced from Anger (1968), by kind permission of the publishers The IAEA.)

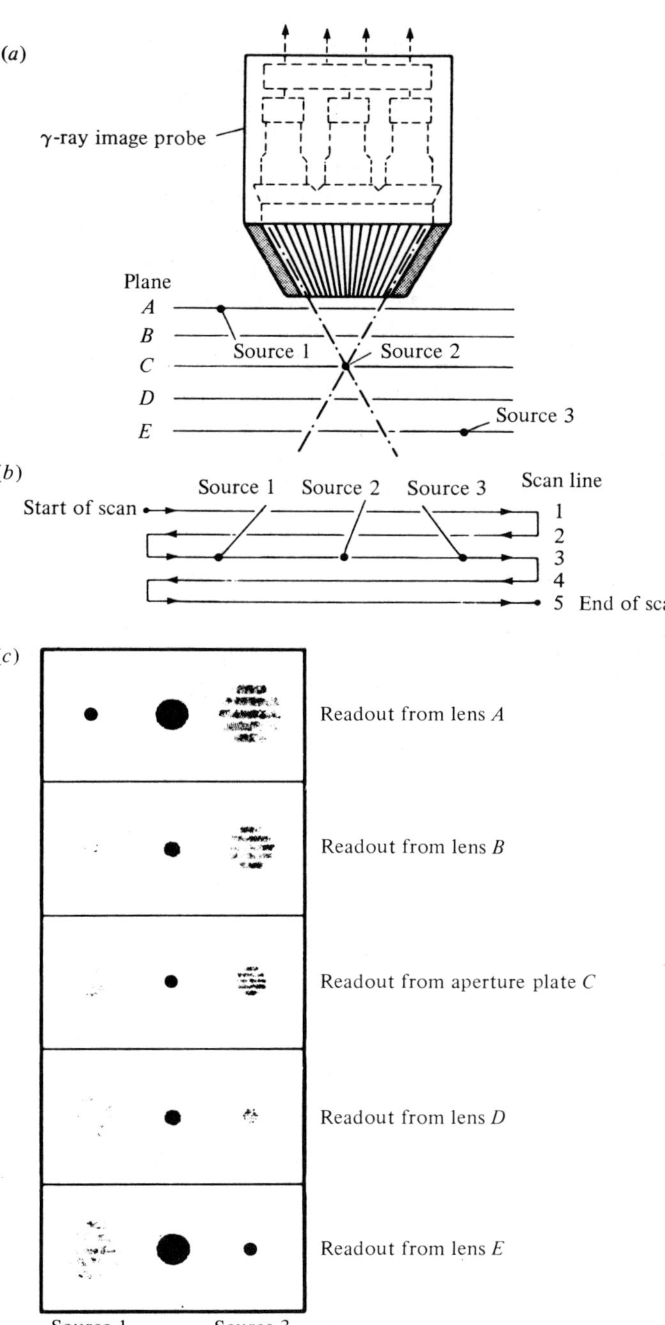

Fig. 7.28. Diagram showing five-plane longitudinal tomogram of three sources at different depths. (*a*) Position of sources; (*b*) movement of detector; (*c*) optical readout. (Reproduced from Anger (1968), by kind permission of the publishers The IAEA.)

and in (*c*) the five-plane scintigram of the three sources. Source 1 is sharply imaged in readout *A*, source 2 in *C*, and source 3 in *E*. This principle has been utilised in the Searle tomographic scanner, a photograph of which is shown in Fig. 7.29(*a*). Twelve simultaneous tomograms of the skeleton, obtained after injection of ^{99m}Tc[EHDP], are shown in Fig. 7.29(*b*). The top six were obtained with the top detector, the extreme right being the most anterior and the others going down towards the mid-plane; the lower six were obtained with the under detector, the extreme left being the most posterior and the others going towards the mid-plane. The way in which different parts of the skeleton are brought into focus is clearly demonstrated.

Transmission computerised transaxial tomography (TCAT) and emission computerised transaxial tomography (ECAT) were referred to in the introduction to this chapter. The basic approach is the same in both, and is the reconstruction, using mathematical techniques, of a tomographic section from a series of one-dimensional projections of an object. TCAT is outside the scope of this book, and discussion will be confined to ECAT systems. It

Fig. 7.29. (*a*) A longitudinal tomographic scanner. (*b*) Simultaneous tomograms of the skeleton produced with equipment shown in (*a*). (Photographs kindly provided by G.D. Searle & Co. Ltd.)

(*a*)

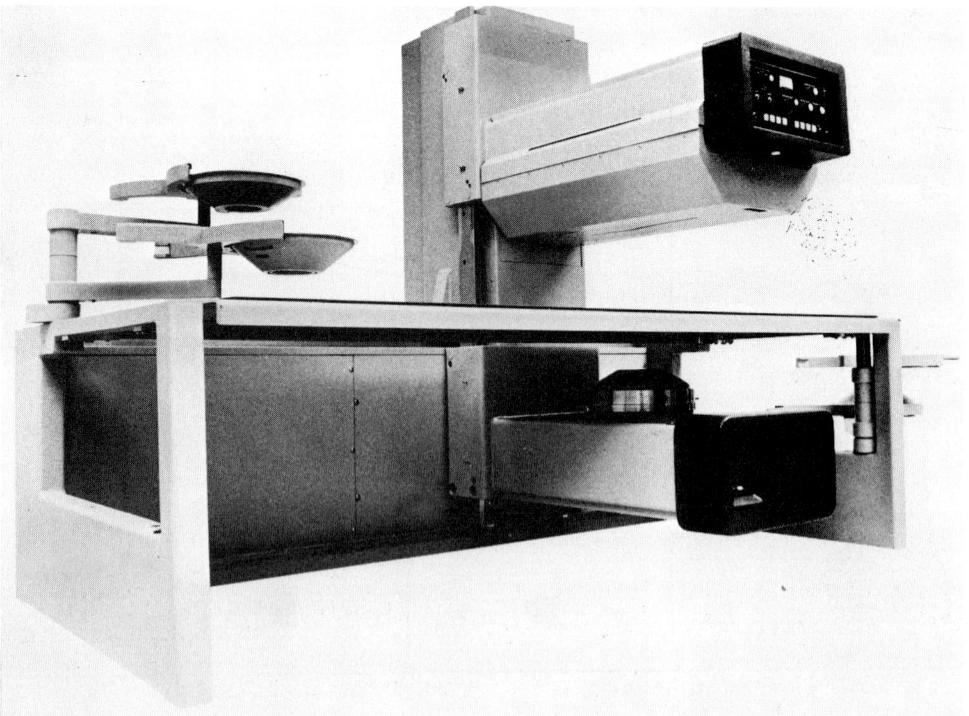

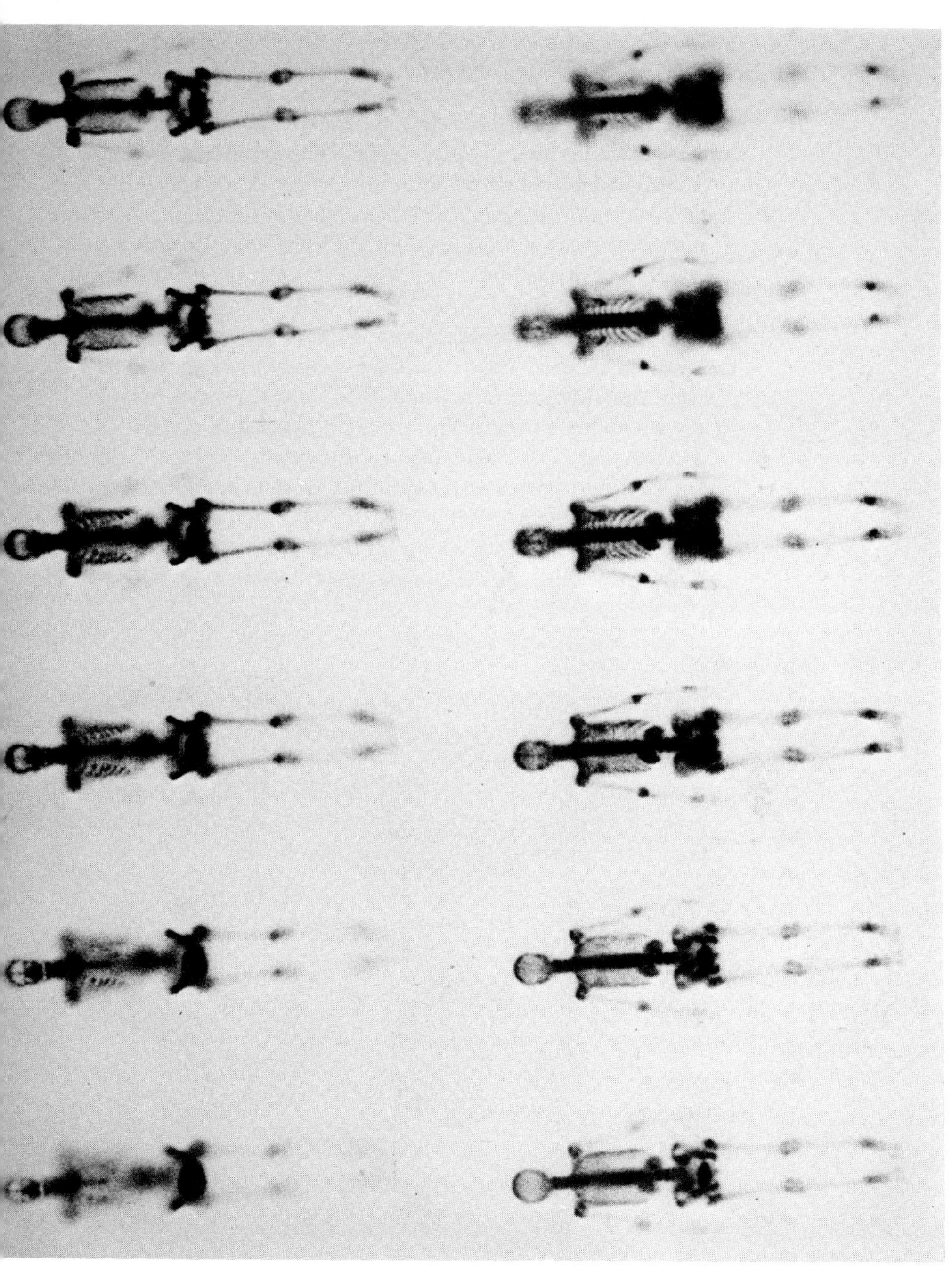

should be appreciated that these procedures produce images of transverse sections of the body, in contrast to those described above which produce longitudinal sections.

ECAT systems fall into two categories: those systems detecting single photons (SP) and those detecting annihilation radiation of positron emitters (annihilation coincidence detectors, ACD). The principle and operation are similar in both; the essential difference is that collimation is achieved in SP by the use of focussed collimators and in ACD by electronic means. SP systems will be considered first.

The principle of an SP system is shown in Fig. 7.30, as set up for brain imaging. The detector is collimated so that only radiation from the transverse plane under investigation is recorded, and there is no unwanted information from other planes. The detector scans one linear pass over the object, collecting data as a series of one-dimensional projections, of sizes determined by the resolution of the collimator. The detector then rotates through a discrete angle, typically 5 degrees, and again scans one linear pass. This is repeated for several angles. Each one-dimensional projection may be considered as a series of elements and, if measurements are made over a sufficient number of angles, the distribution of radionuclide density within the section may be determined. The reconstruction of the image from its projections may be carried out by a variety of mathematical processes, all of considerable complexity, generally performed by a computer; the theory is beyond the scope of this book. A review of these methods is presented by Brooks & Di Chiro (1976). However, it will be evident from the above discussion that certain requirements must be

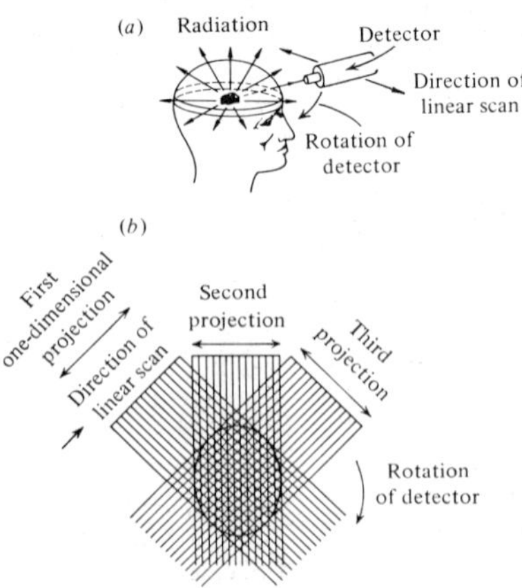

Fig. 7.30. Diagram showing the principle of the ECAT (SP) system. (*a*) The detector scanning a linear pass over one transverse section of the head. (*b*) the one-dimensional projections of the section, obtained from three different angles as the detector rotates. (Reproduced from Brooks & De Chiro (1976), by kind permission of the publishers The Institute of Physics.)

met. These are firstly that the collimation should provide sharp and uniform resolution, and also uniform response (efficiency) throughout the depth of the object, secondly that there must be accurate correction for absorption of radiation within the object, and thirdly that the detector system must have high efficiency to provide good statistics. To date the SP system has been used, mainly in brain imaging, by Kuhl (Kuhl *et al.*, 1977), Mallard & W.I. Keyes (1975), Jaszczak *et al.* (1977) and J.W. Keyes *et al.* (1977). This principle is utilised in the J & P Tomoscanner, which incorporates two opposing detectors each with a focussed collimator. Fig. 7.31(*a*) shows the system set up as for conventional anterior–posterior scanning, and (*b*) demonstrates the tomographic movement by showing four superimposed photographs of the frame and two detectors, as it rotates from 0 to 45, 90 and 135 degrees. Fig. 7.32 shows: in (*a*) and (*b*) the conventional static lateral and anterior images of a brain, which show no abnormality, and in (*c*) and (*d*) the transverse tomograms taken at the levels indicated by the arrows in (*a*). The abnormality in (*c*) is clearly visible. These systems have been found particularly useful in investigating abnormalities at the base of the brain.

SP tomography may also be achieved with a gamma camera system (Jaszczak *et al.*, 1977; Keyes *et al.*, 1977), although there are disadvantages compared with the focussed detector system. The system developed by Jaszczak *et al.* (1977) is shown in

Fig. 7.31. (*a*) J & P tomographic scanner in static mode. (*b*) J & P tomographic scanner demonstrating rotation. (Photographs kindly provided by J. & P. Engineering Ltd.)

(*a*)

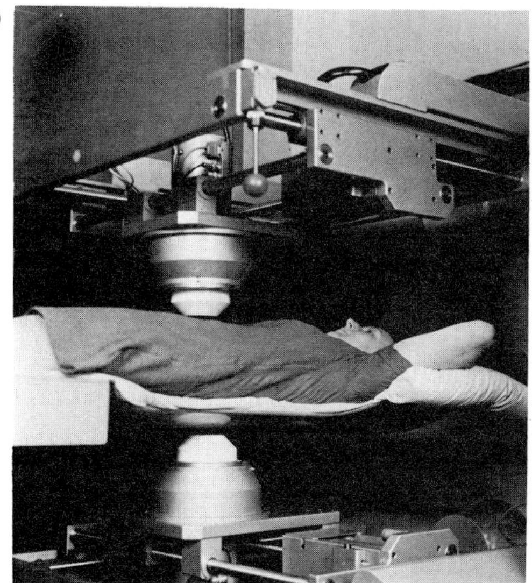

(*b*)

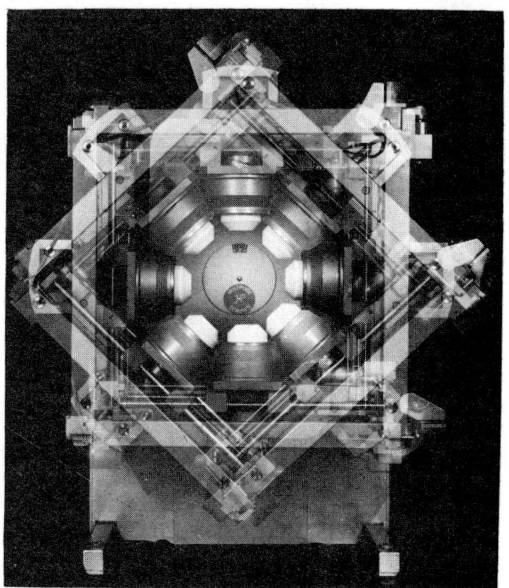

Fig. 7.32. (*a*) and (*b*). Conventional lateral and anterior images of brain. (*c*) and (*d*) transverse tomograms of sections indicated by arrows in (*a*). (Photographs kindly provided by J. & P. Engineering Ltd.)

(*a*)

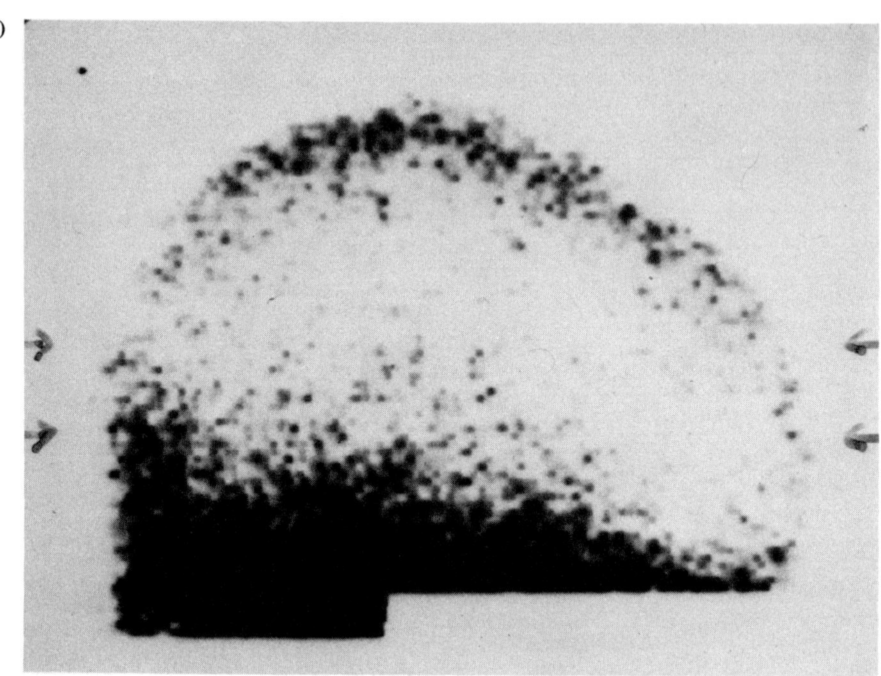

(*c*)

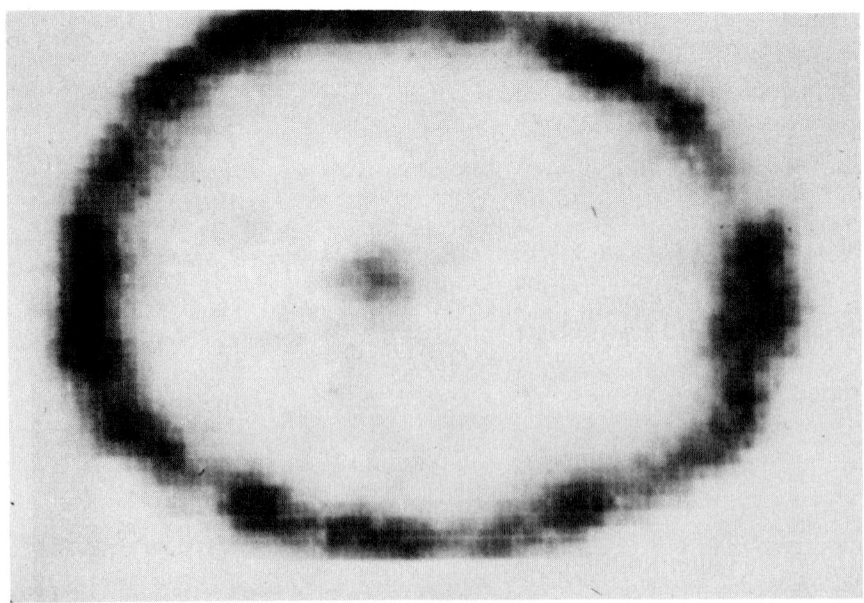

(b)

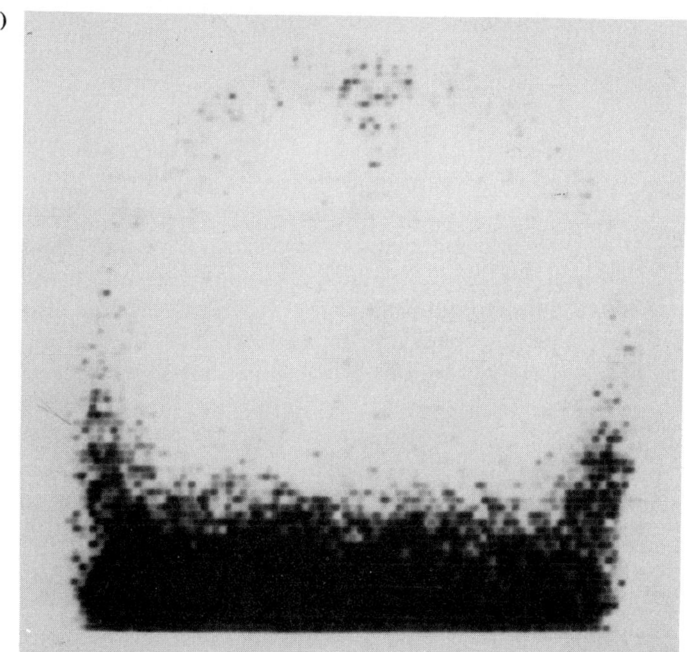

(d)

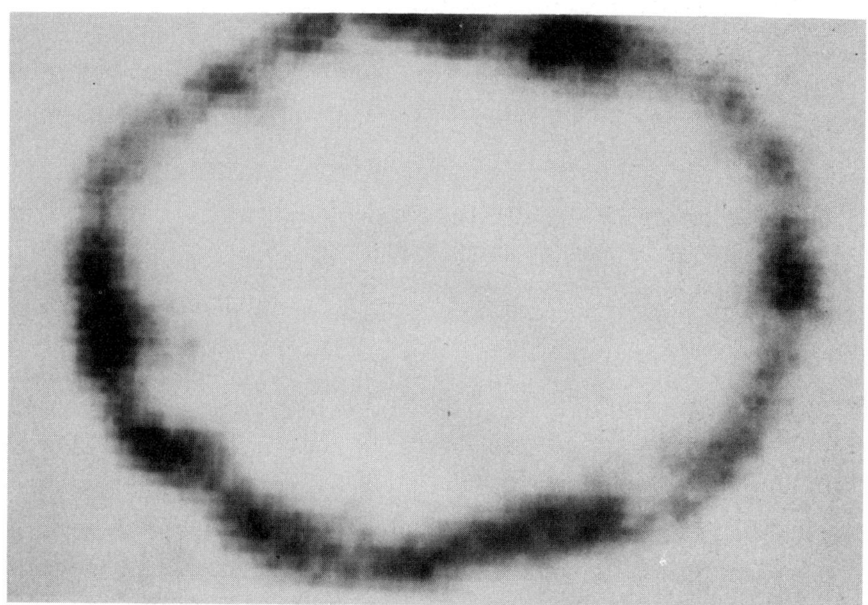

Fig. 7.33. For any one camera position, data are collected simultaneously for one-dimensional projections over the whole object so that linear scanning is unnecessary. The detector makes a single 360-degree revolution about the object, and data are recorded along with a detector-orientation signal at discrete intervals, for example every 4 degrees. It is then possible to select the data for any particular section, and typically nine cross-sections of the brain can be reconstructed (Fig. 7.34). The camera detector system does not conform to the requirements specified above, in that both resolution and response deteriorate with depth. However, if the geometric mean response is used from two opposing views, the response is much improved and approximates to the requirements, particularly for relatively small objects such as the head. By using a 360-degree rotation the geometric mean response can be obtained. The usefulness of this system is illustrated in Fig. 7.35, which clearly demonstrates a craniopharyngioma in the tomogram that is not seen in the conventional

Fig. 7.33. Photograph of gamma camera ECAT (SP) system. (Reproduced from Jaszczak *et al.* (1977), by kind permission of the publishers The Society of Nuclear Medicine.)

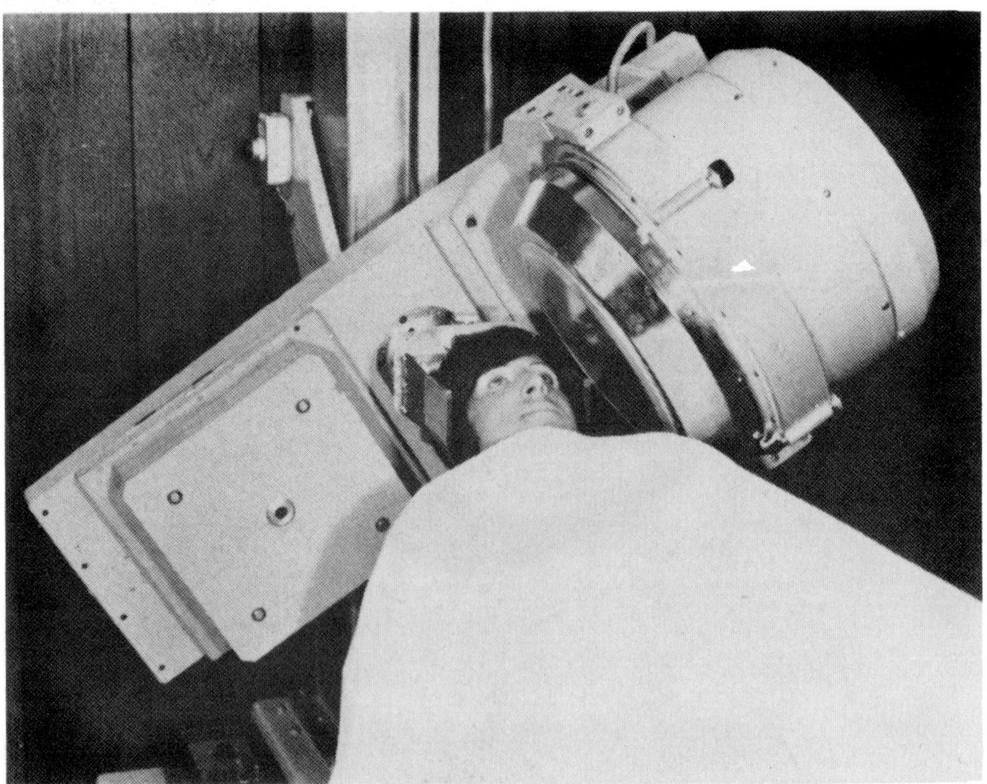

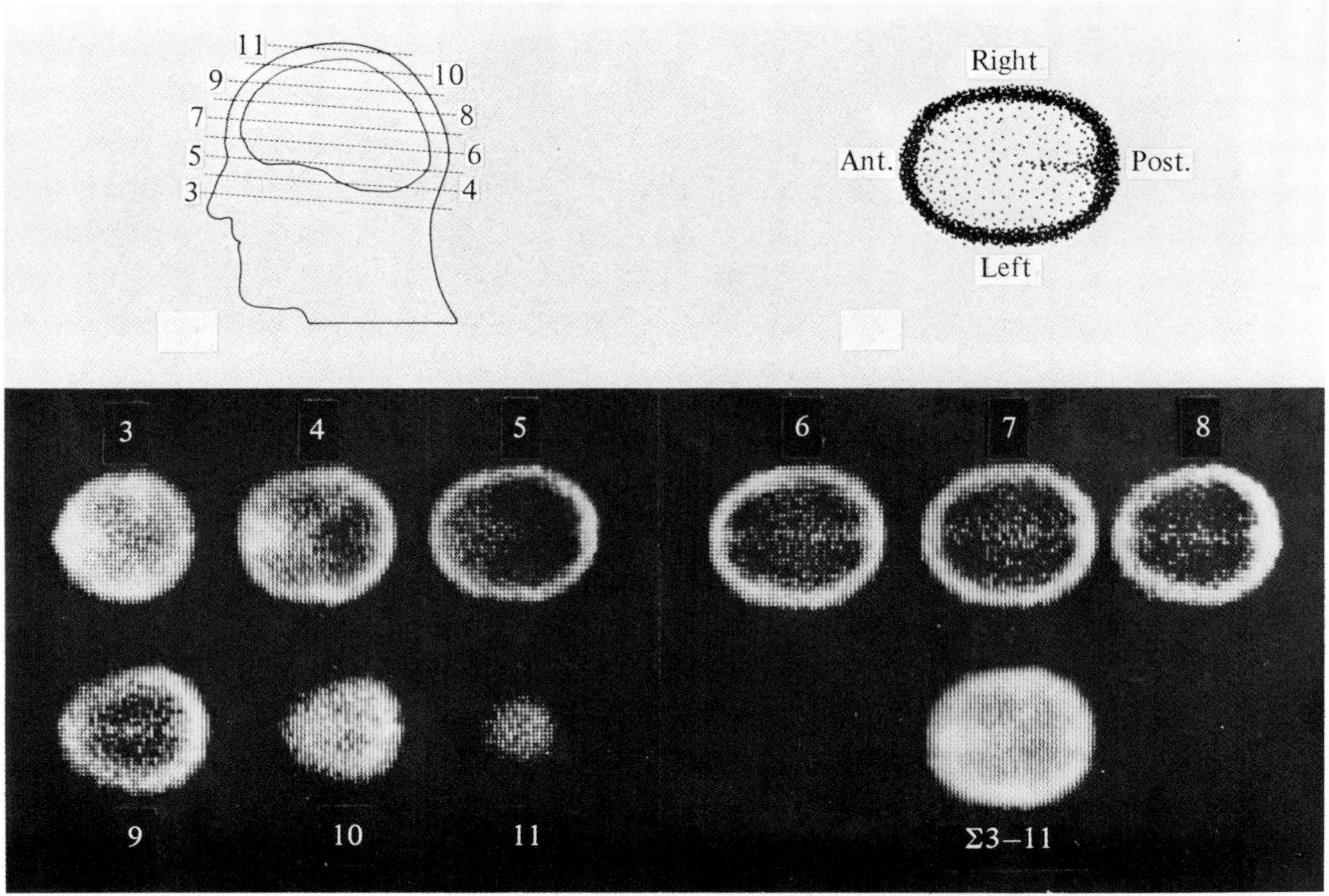

Fig. 7.34. Nine simultaneous transverse tomograms obtained with equipment shown in Fig. 7.33. (Reproduced from Jaszczak *et al.* (1977), by kind permission of the publishers The Society of Nuclear Medicine.)

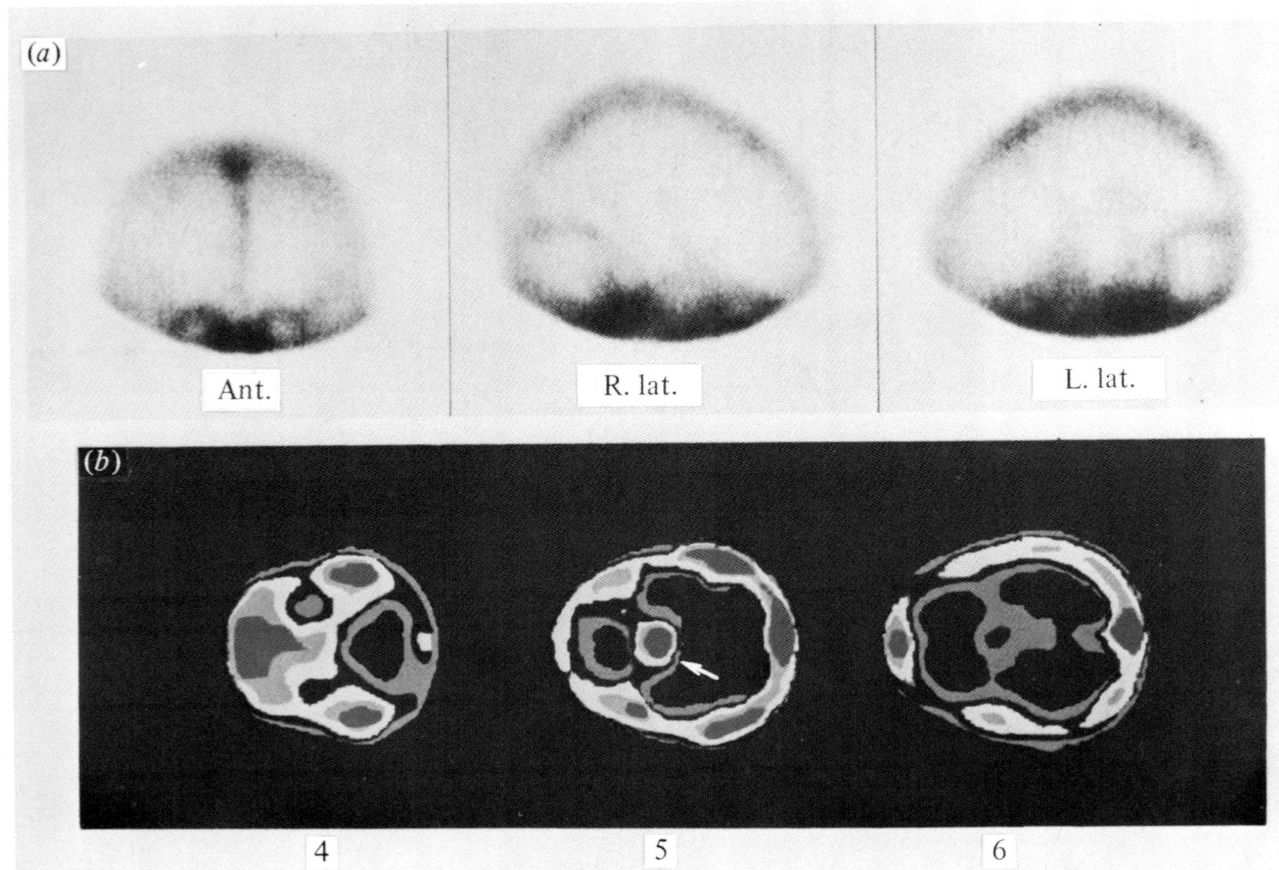

Fig. 7.35. (*a*) Conventional gamma camera views of brain. (*b*) transverse tomograms obtained with equipment shown in Fig. 7.33, demonstrating a craniopharyngioma (arrowed) not seen in the conventional views. (Reproduced from Jaszczak *et al.* (1977), by kind permission of the publishers The Society of Nuclear Medicine.)

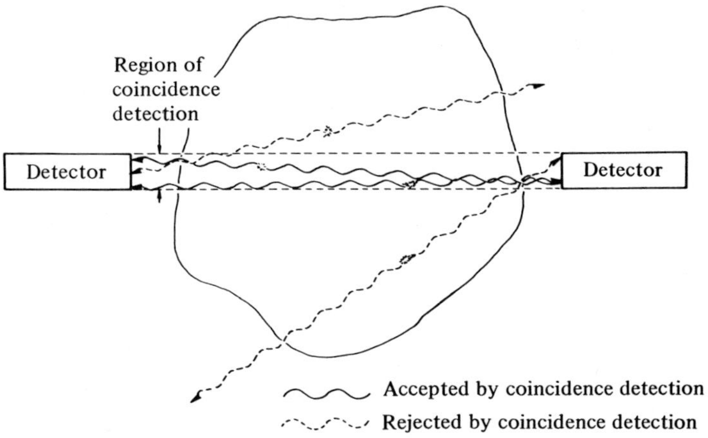

Region of coincidence detection
Detector
Detector
Accepted by coincidence detection
Rejected by coincidence detection

Fig. 7.36. Diagram showing principle of ECAT (ACD) systems. (Reproduced from Phelps *et al.* (1975), by kind permission of the publishers The Society of Nuclear Medicine.)

Interdata model 70 computer
Interface
AMP
PHA
Fast coinci-dence circuit
PHA
AMP
Pre-amplifier
5 cm × 5 cm NaI crystal
Δ₁
Δ₂
Δ = displacement off centre
Δ₃

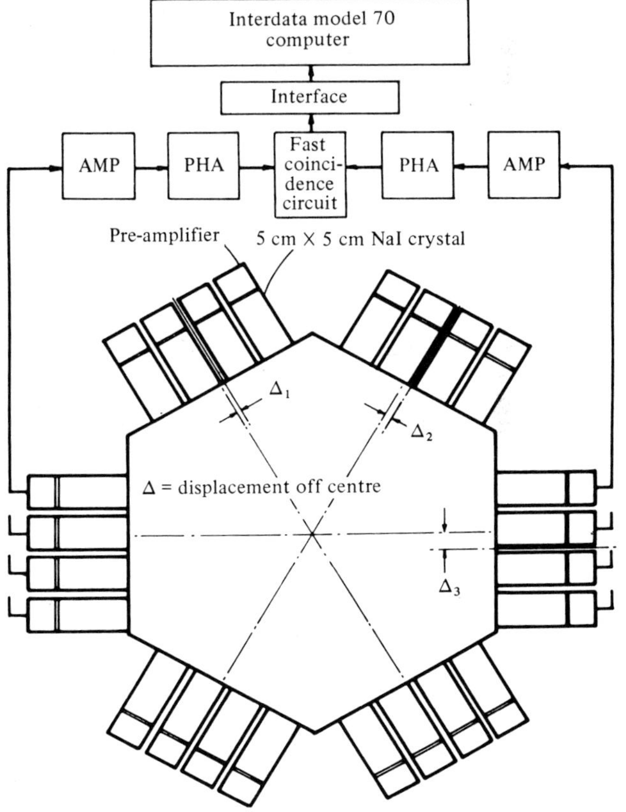

Fig. 7.37. Schematic illustration of prototype PETT. (Reproduced from Phelps *et al.* (1975), by kind permission of the publishers, The Society of Nuclear Medicine.)

Fig. 7.38. The Ortec ECAT system. (Reproduced from Phelps *et al.* (1977), by kind permission of the publishers The IAEA.)

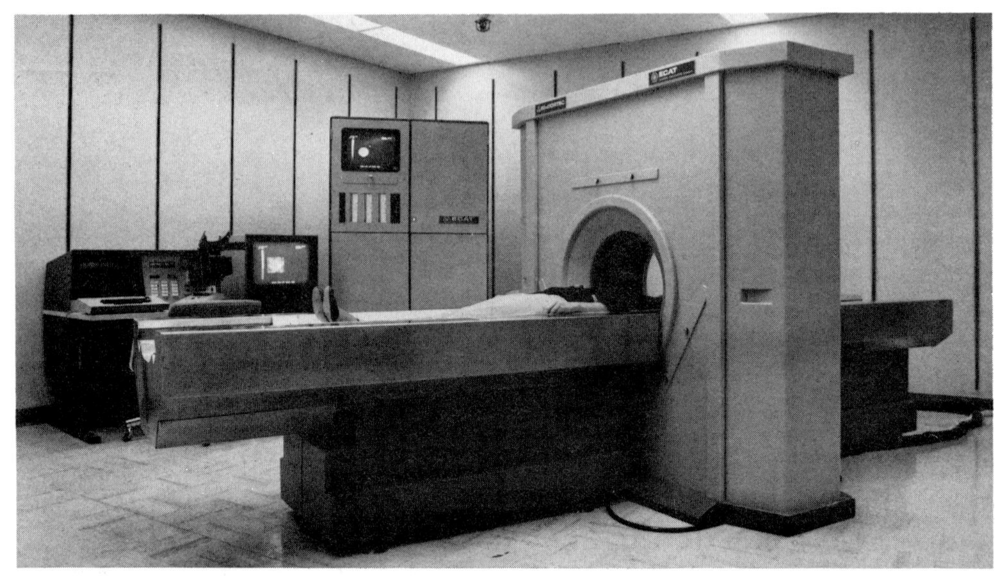

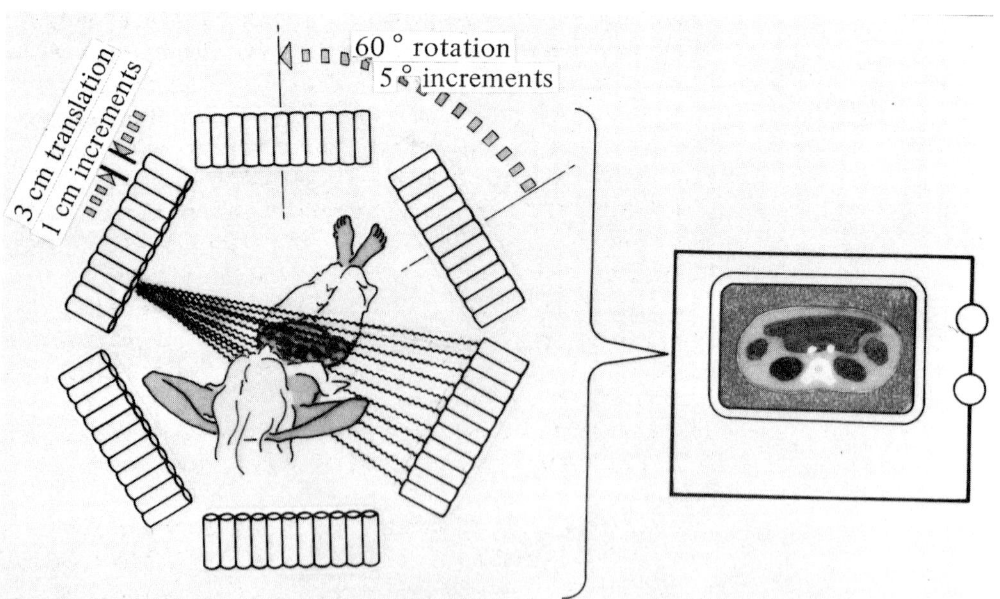

Fig. 7.39. Schematic illustration of Ortec ECAT system. (Reproduced from Phelps *et al.* (1977), by kind permission of the publishers the IAEA.)

gamma camera view.

Many ECAT ACD systems have been designed to detect annihilation radiation from positron-emitting radionuclides. As explained above, the essential difference from the SP systems is that the collimation is obtained electronically by the coincidence system, as demonstrated in Fig. 7.36, instead of physically by using a focussed collimator. It will be observed that the electronic collimation conforms to the requirements given for SP systems. The detectors used may be hexagonal scanners, dual-head multi-crystal scanners, dual-head single-crystal or multi-crystal cameras.

A prototype positron-emission transaxial tomograph (PETT) has been developed at St Louis by Phelps *et al.* (1975) and produced commercially by Ortec Inc. The detection system of the prototype is shown schematically in Fig. 7.37. It consists of 24 NaI detectors placed in a hexagonal array, four to a side. The four detectors on one bank are in coincidence with the four detectors on the opposite bank. In operation, the object is placed at the centre of the 24-detector system, which is rotated under computer control. Coincidence data from the 12 pairs of detectors are recorded every 7.5 degrees through a full 360 degree rotation of the object under study. The prototype was used to evaluate the performance of such a system. The Ortec ECAT system is shown in Fig. 7.38; it consists of a hexagonal array of 66 NaI detectors in which 11 detectors on one bank are in coincidence with all 11 detectors on the opposing bank. This results in 121 lines of response between detector banks, with a total of 363 for the system (Fig. 7.39). One of the unique features of ACD is that the detector can record and position events with a fan beam geometry, unlike collimated detectors which are limited to a straight-ahead field of view. During operation the patient is positioned at the centre of the detector array. All six banks synchronously perform linear scans over 3 cm, the gantry rotates typically through 5 degrees, linear scan motion is reversed, and the process is repeated until a total rotation of 60 degrees is achieved.

An example of results obtained with the Ortec system is shown in Fig. 7.40 (Phelps, Hoffman & Kuhl, 1977). $^{13}NH_3$ was injected intravenously and tomographic scans were carried out from 1 cm below the orbito-meatal line to the top of the brain. $^{13}NH_3$ distributes through the tissue in proportion to the blood perfusion, diffuses from the blood at the capillary level, and is retained in the tissues by metabolism into amino acids, with a tissue clearance half-time of 50 to 60 minutes. The authors conclude that the tomographic $^{13}NH_3$ images appear to represent the perfusion distribution, since they found excellent agreement between the uptake of $^{13}NH_3$ in cerebellum, vermus, brain stem, superficial cortex and subcortical white matter, the measured values of capillary densities in human subjects, and autoradiographic studies of cerebral blood flow in cats.

The purpose of ECAT and the relative merits of SP and ACD systems have been discussed by Phelps (1977). SP systems have been used mainly for brain studies because of the problems of maintaining a relative constant resolution with depth, and of attenuation corrections; ACD systems, on the other hand, provide resolution and high contrast that is depth-independent, and attenuation is correctable by a near exact technique. SP systems do have the great advantage though that they can be used with radiopharmaceuticals labelled with ^{99m}Tc and the commercially available nuclides, whereas ACD systems require an on-site accelerator for studies using the positron emitters ^{11}C, ^{13}N and ^{15}O. The importance of ECAT is its capability of sectioning an organ tomographically with high resolution and accuracy, into a map of quantitative tracer concentration. It performs physiologic or function tomography, whereas TCAT performs morphological tomography.

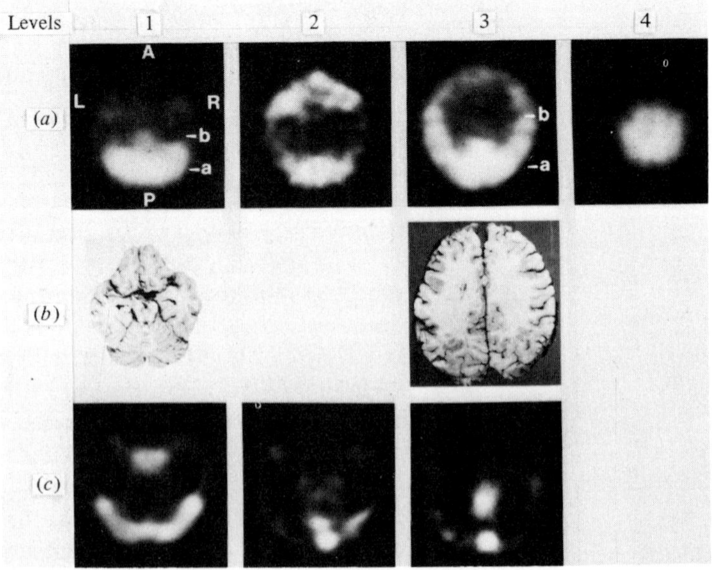

Fig. 7.40. Results obtained with Ortec ECAT system. Transverse sections of the brain showing (*a*) concentration of $^{13}NH_3$, (*b*) corresponding anatomical section (*c*) concentration of ^{11}CO. (Reproduced from Phelps *et al.* (1977), by kind permission of the publishers the IAEA.)

References

Anger, H.O. (1969). Multiplane tomographic gamma-ray scanner. In *Medical Radioisotope Scintigraphy*, vol. 1, pp. 200–13. Vienna: International Atomic Energy Agency.

Atkins, F.B., Beck, R.N., Hoffer, P.B. & Palmer, D. (1977). Dependence of optimum baseline setting on scatter fraction and detector response function. (SM-210/76). In *Medical Radionuclide Imaging*, vol. 1, pp. 101–18. Vienna: International Atomic Energy Avency.

Bender, M.A. & Blau, M. (1963). The autofluoroscope. *Nucleonics* **21**, 52–6.

Brooks, R.A. & Di Chiro, G. (1976). Principles of computer assisted tomography (CAT) in radiographic and radioisotopic imaging. *Phys. Med. Biol.* **21**, 690–732.

Ell, P.J., Al-Eid, M., Lui, D., Pearce, P.C., Elliott, A.T. & Brown, N.J.G. (1977). High-quality, high throughput, early whole-body bone scanning. *Nucl. Med.* **16**(5), 238–40.

HPA (1977). *The Theory, Specification and Testing of Anger-type Gamma Cameras.* London: Hospital Physicists' Association, Radionuclide Topic Group.

Hounsfield, G.N. (1973). Computerised transverse axial scanning (tomography). I: Description of system. *B. J. Radiol.* **46**, 1016–47.

IEC (1978). Draft: *Characteristics and Test Conditions of Radionuclide Imaging Devices.* IEC Document 62C (Secretariat) 13. London: British Standards Institution (Ref. BSI 78/32345).

Jaszczak, R.J., Murphy, P.H., Huard, D. & Burdine, J.A. (1977). Radionuclide emission computed tomography of the head with ^{99m}Tc and a scintillation camera. *J. Nucl. Med.* **18**, 373–80.

Keyes, J.W. Jr, Orlandea, N., Heetderks, W.J., Leonard, P.F. & Roger, W.L. (1977). The Humongotron – a scintillation camera transaxial tomograph. *J. Nucl. Med.* **18**, 381–7.

Kuhl, D.E. & Edwards, R.Q. (1963). Image separation scanning. *Radiology*, **117**, 653–62.

Kuhl, D.E., Hoffman, E.J., Phelps, M.E. & Ricci, A. (1977). Design and application of Mark IV Scanning System for radionuclide computed tomography of the brain. In *Medical Radionuclide Imaging*, vol. 1, pp. 309–18. Vienna: International Atomic Energy Agency.

Lange, D., Hermann, H.J., Wetzel, E. & Schenck, P. (1977). Critical parameters to estimate the use of a scintillation camera in high dose dynamic studies. In *Medical Radionuclide Imaging*, vol. 1, pp. 85–100. Vienna: International Atomic Energy Agency.

Lunt, R. (1978). *Handbook of Ultrasonic B-Scanning in Medicine. Techniques of Measurement in Medicine 1.* Cambridge University Press.

Macintyre, W.J., Fedoruk, S.O., Harris, C.C., Kuhl, D.E. & Mallard, J.R. (1969). Sensitivity and resolution in radioisotope scanning. In *Medical Radioisotope Scintigraphy*, vol. 1, pp. 391–435. Vienna: International Atomic Energy Agency.

Mallard, J. (1972). The radionuclide imaging process and factors influencing the choice of an instrument for brain scanning. In *Progress in Nuclear Medicine*, vol. 1, p. 1. Baltimore/Basel: Karger/University Park Press.

Mallard, J. & Keyes, W.I. (1975). The technique and use of isotope transverse section tomography. In *The New Image in Tomography*, pp. 76–88. Amsterdam: Excerpta Medica.

Myers, M.J., Keyes, W.I. & Mallard, J.R. (1973). An analysis of tomographic scanning systems. In *Medical Radioisotope Scintigraphy*, vol. 1, pp. 331–45. Vienna: International Atomic Energy Agency.

Phelps, M.E. (1977). What is the purpose of emission computed tomography in nuclear medicine? *J. Nucl. Med.* **18**, 399–402.

Phelps, M.E., Hoffman, E.J. & Kuhl, D.E. (1977). Physiologic tomography (PT) – a new approach to in-vivo measure of metabolism and physiological function. In *Medical Radionuclide Imaging*, vol. 1, pp. 233–51. Vienna: International Atomic Energy Agency.

Phelps, M.E., Hoffman, E.J., Mullani, N.A. & Ter Pogossian, M.M. (1975). Application of annihilation coincidence detection to transaxial reconstruction tomography. *J. Nucl. Med.* **16**, 210–24.

Rose, A. (1957). Quantum effects in human vision. In *Advances in Biological and Medical Physics*, vol. 5, p. 211. New York & London: Academic Press.

Smith, E.M. & Katchie, L. Jr (1969). Multifunction digital research scanning system (SM-108/85). In *Medical Radioisotope Scintigraphy*, pp. 187–201. Vienna: International Atomic Energy Agency.

Sorenson, J.A. (1976). Methods of correcting Anger camera deadtime losses. *J. Nucl. Med.* **17**, 137–41.

Todd-Pokropek, A., Erbsmann, F. & Soussaline, F. (1977). The non-uniformity of imaging devices and its impact in quantitative studies (SM-210/154). In *Medical Radionuclide Imaging*, vol. 1, pp. 67–82. Vienna: International Atomic Energy Agency.

USDHEW (1977). *Measurements of the Performance Parameters of Gamma Cameras*, part 1. HEW Publication (FDA) 78-8049. Rockville: United States Department of Health, Education and Welfare.

Verdon, T.A. & Allen, F.H. (1969). Dynapix: a new concept in rapid rectilinear scanning (SM-108/84). In *Medical Radioisotope Scintigraphy*, pp. 177–84. Vienna: International Atomic Energy Agency.

Woodrough, R.E. (1979). *Medical Infra-Red Thermography: Principles and Practice.* Cambridge University Press (in preparation).

8. Dynamic measurement of uptake

Introduction

Dynamic studies are those in which radioactivity in the body is measured as a function of time. They cover a wide range of techniques and include simple uptake measurements carried out at intervals using a single-probe, or multi-probe system, measurements on a whole-body counter, sophisticated methods using gamma cameras and fast data collection, and emission computed tomography with positron emitters. These will be considered in turn.

Single-probe and multi-probe measurements

The main problem with uptake measurements using a single probe is to ensure that positioning over the organ is accurate. If measurements are to be continued over several days, for example thyroid uptake measurements, or splenic and liver uptake in red cell survival studies, then in addition the position must be reproducible. Sometimes the organ can be located before starting the study and this should be done when possible. For example, the spleen and liver can be located with a [^{99m}Tc] antimony sulphide colloid scan, and surface markings made prior to a red cell survival study; it is most easily done on a rectilinear scanner, by positioning the detector over the region of interest. Collimation is important; ideally the collimator should be designed so that only the organ of interest is viewed by the detector and the detector response is constant and highly efficient for all points in the organ. In practice this is never achieved, and the compromise of the so-called flat-field collimator is used; this has a fairly uniform response within its field of view at any given depth, and the response falls off sharply at the edges. The response falls off with depth mainly as a result of absorption, and the collimator design must ensure adequate response at the required depth. If the measurements are to be continued over a period of days it is also important to ensure consistency of performance of the equipment, and standard sources should be counted before and after each measurement; if these show significant changes in sensitivity appropriate corrections should be applied.

Dynamic studies are usually concerned with changes in uptake, but it is often required to determine the absolute uptake or the relative uptake in two or more organs. There are several problems. Firstly, there is usually a background due to activity in tissue other than the organ of interest, most commonly in the blood but sometimes in other adjacent organs. Background subtraction techniques are used to correct for this and sometimes dual-isotope techniques are useful. Another difficulty arises from absorption and scattering of the radiation emitted from the organ, both in the organ itself and in the overlying tissue. By making measurements on phantoms in a scattering medium, with the physical characteristics of the former as close as possible to those of the organ in question, it is possible to allow for scattering and absorption and to estimate absolute uptake. Occasionally it is possible to confirm these estimates by measurements on specimens obtained at operation.

Probe renography

This is probably the most widely used dynamic technique involving the use of probes and can be used to illustrate the principles involved. The investigation is aimed at assessing individual kidney

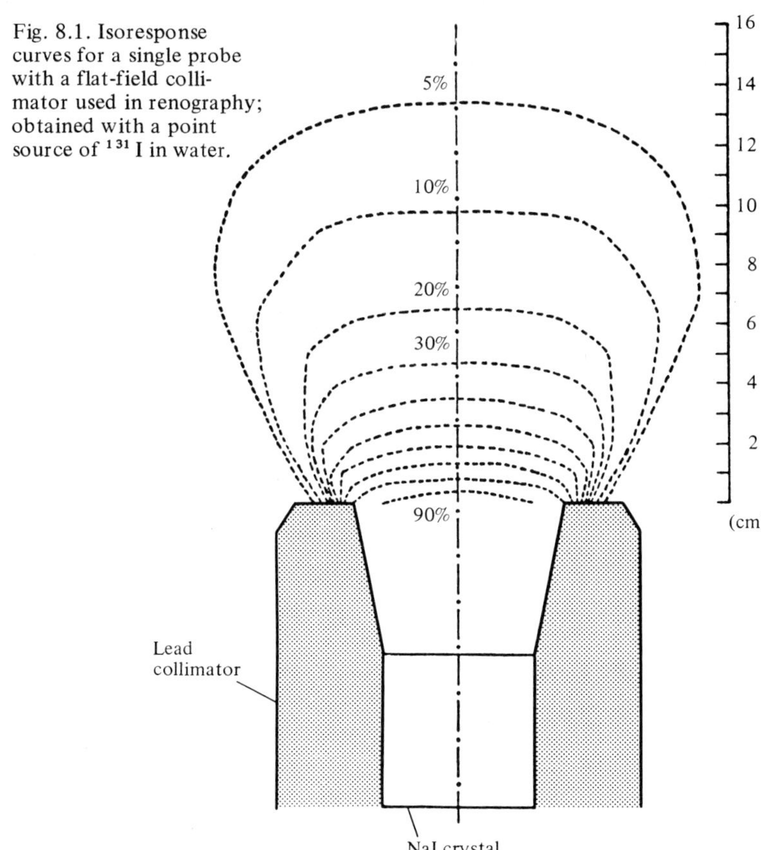

Fig. 8.1. Isoresponse curves for a single probe with a flat-field collimator used in renography; obtained with a point source of ^{131}I in water.

function by determining the uptake of radioactive iodo-orthohippuric acid, known as hippuran, by the kidneys and its subsequent excretion. To achieve this, two scintillation probes are centred one over each kidney and a third detector is placed over the sub-clavicular area; [^{131}I]hippuran is injected and continuous measurements are made for a period of 20 to 30 minutes.

Equipment. Three scintillation probes are needed, each with a NaI crystal of 5 cm diameter and thickness, and a flat-field circular or elliptical collimator. The field of view of the collimator at 6 cm depth, which is the average depth of the kidney, should have a diameter of 9 cm, to cover the average kidney. Fig. 8.1 shows the isoresponse curves of a typical system to a point source of ^{131}I in water. The electronic system is as described in Chapter 3, incorporating a charge-sensitive pre-amplifier and pulse-height analyser (PHA) for each probe, and either a ratemeter to record count-rate or a scaling unit. The output from each probe may be taken from the ratemeter to a multichannel rectilinear chart recorder to provide the type of display shown in Fig. 8.2(*a*) and (*b*). Alternatively, or additionally, if digital data are required the output from the scaling unit may be punched out on to paper tape in computer-compatible form.

Positioning. If the investigation is being used as a screening test the position of the kidneys may be located using standard anatomical landmarks. If greater accuracy is required they should be localised by an erect radiograph taken with lead markers *in situ*, using contrast material if necessary, or by imaging after an injection of ^{99m}Tc-labelled DTPA (see Table 5.3). The sub-clavicular positioning is not critical, since this is used only as a vascular area to indicate the changes in blood activity. It is important that the patient is comfortable so that there is no movement during the period of measurement.

Blood background. It is evident that the two counters positioned over the kidneys will detect radiation arising not only from the kidneys but also from the circulating blood which is in the field of view, so that the curve recorded will be a combination of blood clearance and kidney uptake and clearance. Although these curves, combined with the blood clearance (sub-clavicular) curve, give a general indication of kidney function (Fig. 8.2*a*), a more meaningful curve is obtained if a correction can be made for the

Fig. 8.2. (*a*) Typical renogram trace obtained with a multichannel rectilinear recorder. Traces on the left are due to [^{131}I]HSA injection. Traces on the right follow the [^{131}I]hippuran injection.

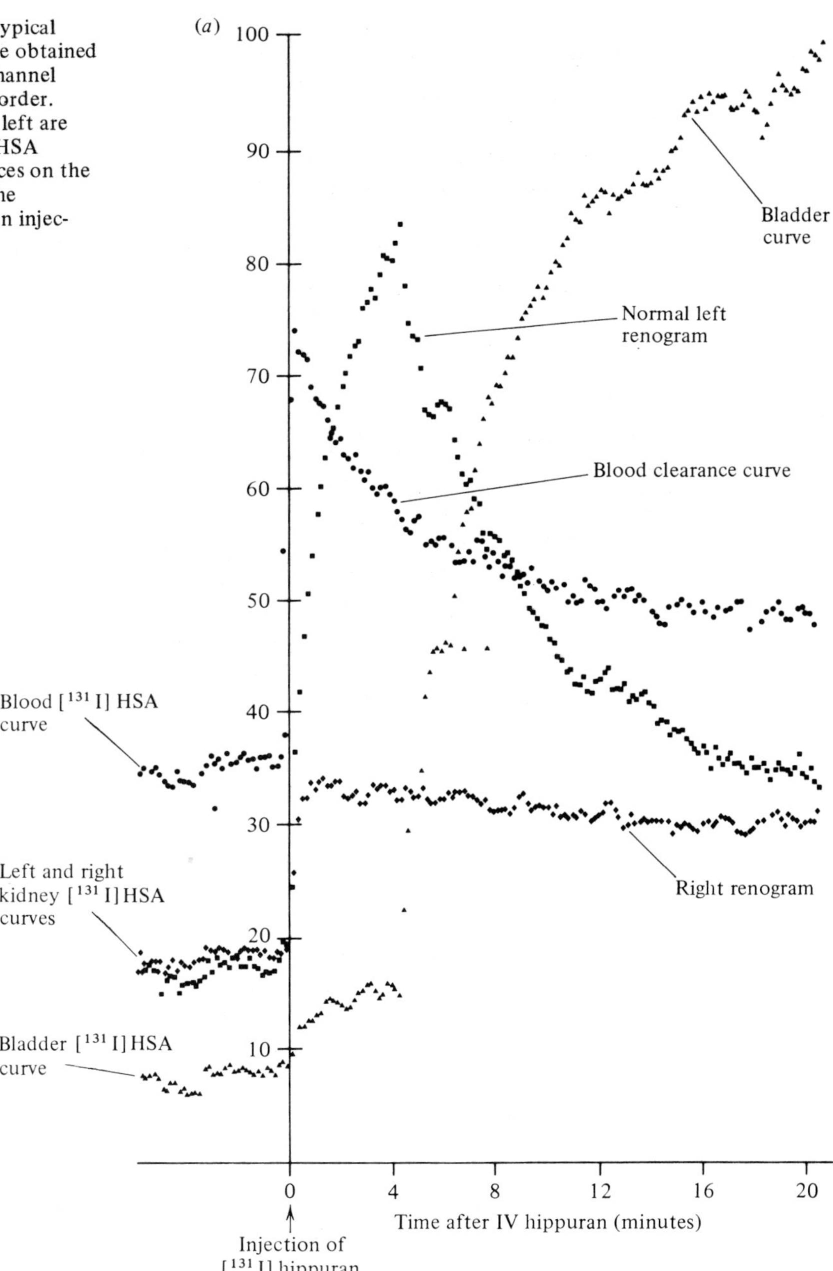

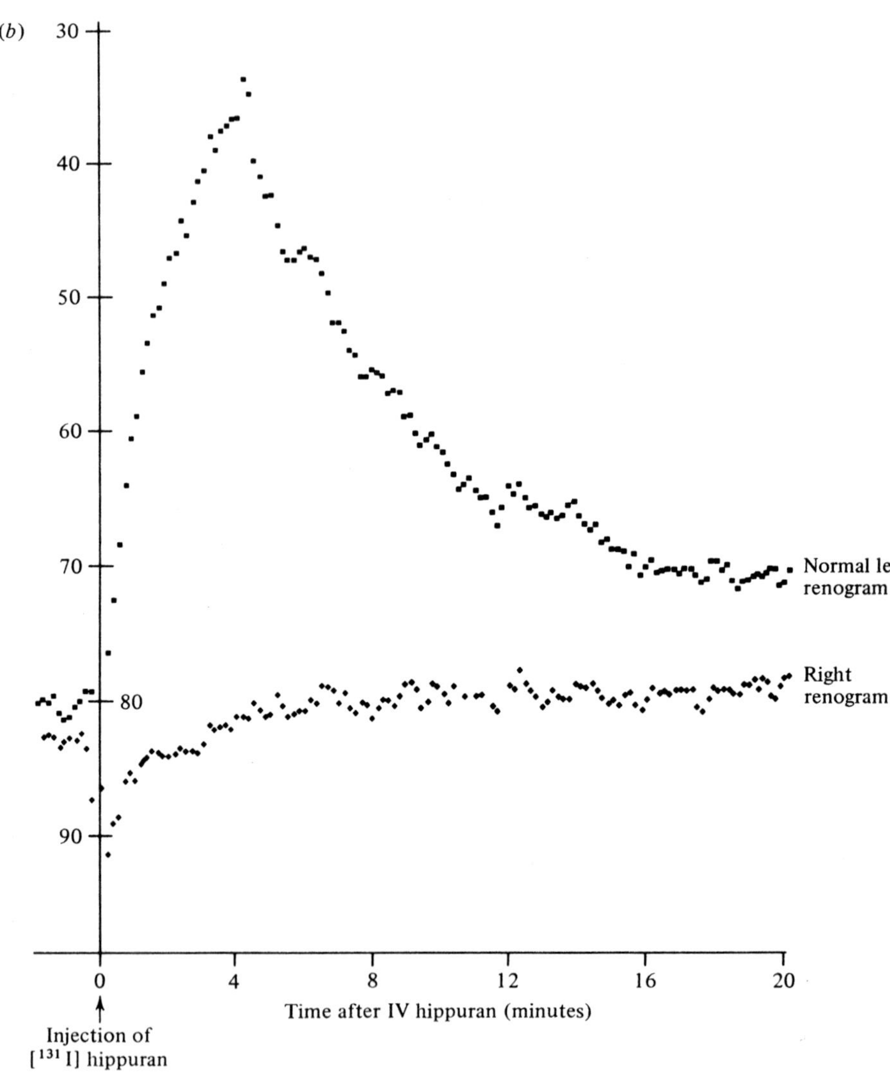

Fig. 8.2. (*b*) Typical renogram trace after analogue blood-background subtraction. Upper curve, normal left renogram; lower curve, right renogram showing poor kidney function. (*c*) The same renogram after digital blood-background subtraction, showing a result similar to (*b*). The right renogram, which is of lower amplitude, has been normalised to a maximum of 50%. (Modified from K.E. Britton & N.J.G. Brown (1971) *Clinical Renography*, by kind permission of the publishers Lloyd-Luke (Medical Books).)

blood activity. This can be done using the sub-clavicular curve, which gives the variation of blood activity with time. A prior injection of a blood-pool agent, e.g. [^{131}I] HSA, is given in order to estimate the blood background contribution in each kidney as a fraction of that recorded in the sub-clavicular detector.

Procedure

(1) Prepare the doses, that is 3 μCi (0.1 MBq) [^{131}I] HSA, and 15 μCi (0.5 MBq) [^{131}I] hippuran according to the master document and take up in separate syringes.

(2) Thyroid blocking is not usually indicated but the appropriate agent should be given to the patient if prescribed.

(3) Ask the patient to empty his bladder.

(4) Mark the position of the kidneys on the patient's back using a skin marker. Get the patient sitting comfortably in the renogram chair, position the two kidney detectors one over each kidney and the third detector over the sub-clavicular area (Fig. 8.3).

(5) Start the electronic equipment to record background counts for 1 or 2 minutes.

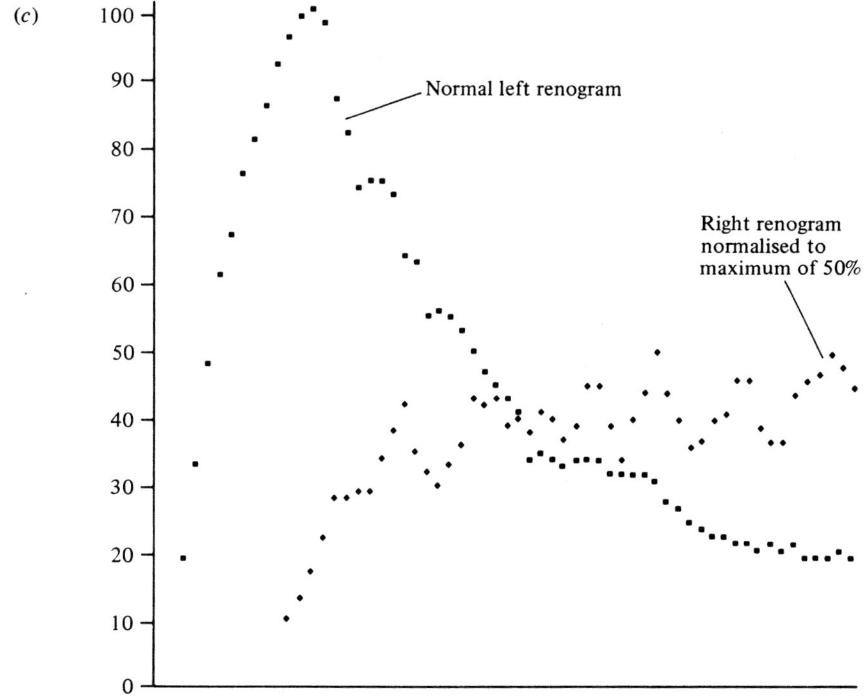

(6) Inject the [^{131}I]HSA and record the two kidney counts and the sub-clavicular counts for 3 to 5 minutes, or until they remain constant. If a subtraction device is available adjust the potentiometer controls so that the resultant kidney counts are zero. This device then subtracts the appropriate constant fraction of the sub-clavicular count from that of each kidney, providing an automatic blood-background subtraction correction (Fig. 8.2*b*).

(7) Inject the [^{131}I]hippuran and record on the chart recorder the three curves described above and also the corrected curves for the left and right kidney, continuing for 20 to 30 minutes.

If the data are being punched out on to paper tape, only the data for the first three curves are needed, because the data can be fed into a computer which is programmed to calculate the blood-background correction and plot the two corrected kidney curves in digital form, as shown in Fig. 8.2(*c*).

(8) If either kidney curve shows slow excretion it is helpful to ask the patient to stand up and walk around for a minute or two. Then re-position accurately and continue measurement for 2 or 3 minutes.

(9) Ask the patient to empty his bladder into a container for collection. Measure the volume passed and calculate the rate of urine flow in millilitres per minute. Sometimes it is helpful to measure the total radioactivity of the specimen.

(10) If an estimate of relative kidney function has been requested the depth of each kidney should be found by ultrasound measurements, in order to correct for differences in depth.

Calculation. The analysis of the results will depend on the information required. For a screening test, visual inspection of the two kidney curves and the sub-clavicular curve (Fig. 8.2*a*) is sufficient. If relative kidney function is required then the blood subtraction correction must be applied, either automatically as described above or by computer processing of the data collected on paper tape.

If the equilibrium counts after [^{131}I]HSA injection are $(K_R)_{HSA}$, $(K_L)_{HSA}$ and $(B)_{HSA}$ respectively, for the right kidney, left kidney and sub-clavicular detector, then the ratio of the blood activity in the right and left kidney regions, respectively, to that in the sub-clavicular region will be $(K_R)_{HSA}/(B)_{HSA}$ and $(K_L)_{HSA}/$

$(B)_{HSA}$. Let these ratios be designated R_R and R_L; for any subsequent activity counts B after injection of [^{131}I]hippuran, the counts recorded by the two kidney detectors due to blood activity will be $R_R B$ and $R_L B$. Subtraction of these from the total kidney counts K_R and K_L will give the counts due to hippuran alone. Thus:

$$(K_R)_{\text{hippuran}} = K_R - R_R B \tag{8.1}$$

$$(K_L)_{\text{hippuran}} = K_L - R_L B \tag{8.2}$$

The counts B include the small activity due to [^{131}I]HSA as well as [^{131}I]hippuran. It should be noted that this method of correction implies that the ratio of the HSA and hippuran spaces is the same in all three fields of view.

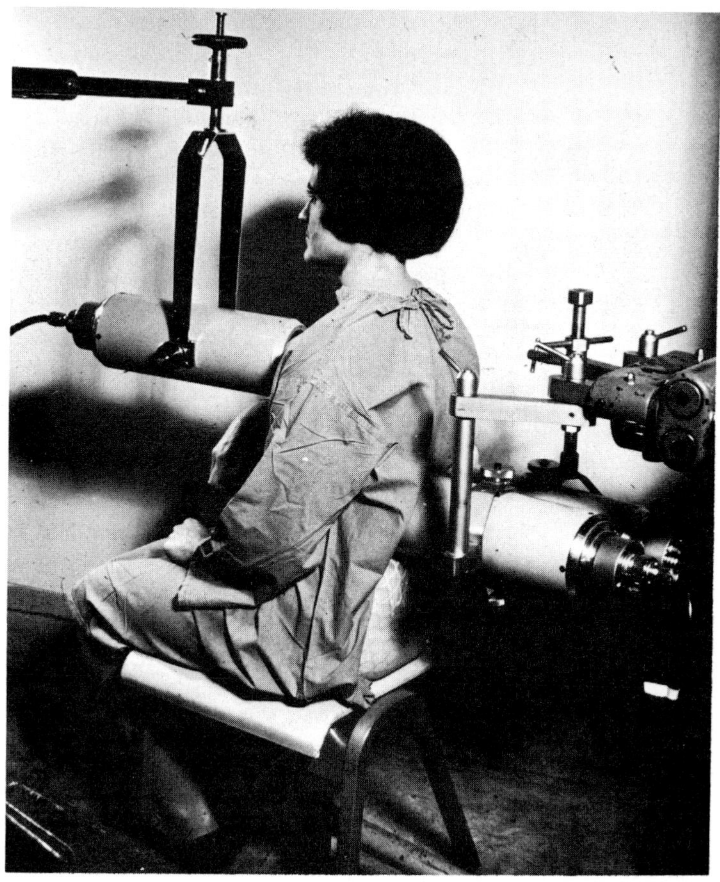

Fig. 8.3. Patient positioned for three-probe renography.

In the corrected curve (Fig. 8.2*b*) the kidney curves should rise from zero to a maximum, which occurs just before the radioactivity starts to leave the kidney and move out of the field of view. The mean ratio of the hippuran counts from the left and right kidneys over this period of time therefore represents their relative uptake function. Since relative function is normally expressed as a percentage of the whole:

$$\text{Right kidney relative function} = \frac{(K_{\mathrm{R}})_{\text{hippuran}}}{(K_{\mathrm{R}})_{\text{hippuran}} + (K_{\mathrm{L}})_{\text{hippuran}}} \qquad (8.3)$$

$$\text{Left kidney relative function} = \frac{(K_{\mathrm{L}})_{\text{hippuran}}}{(K_{\mathrm{R}})_{\text{hippuran}} + (K_{\mathrm{L}})_{\text{hippuran}}} \qquad (8.4)$$

These values may be obtained directly from the chart recorder graph or by computer calculation from the paper tape data. If ultrasound depth measurements are available the appropriate depth correction is made. The paper tape data may be further used for deconvolution techniques. These will be discussed later in this chapter.

Whole-body counters

Whole-body counters, as the name implies, are used to investigate the absorption and retention of radiopharmaceuticals, that is to measure the total activity in the body. There is a wide variety in design, but all aim to achieve the essential feature, which is uniformity of response to a source anywhere in the body. This is never completely realised and the response is evidently dependent not only on the relative geometry between the body and detectors but also on the absorption and scattering of the emitted radiation within the body, and these vary with the energy of the radiation.

A widely used system is the shadow-shield, and a typical set-up is shown in Fig. 8.4. The detecting system consists of four large (15 cm diameter) NaI crystals, each with its PM tube, arranged in a plane perpendicular to the couch on which the patient lies. Two detectors are above and two below the couch. Thus they view a transverse section of the body, and the width of that section is determined by two collimator slits, one above and one below the patient. The couch has a motor drive which can move it, at pre-selected constant speed, along its length so that each transverse section of the body is presented in turn to the

NaI scintillation detector assembly

Stainless steel shielding

Stainless steel collimator slits

Moving couch

Fig. 8.4. Drawing of a shadow-shield whole-body counter. (Modified from the drawing by Nuclear Enterprises Ltd, with their kind permission.)

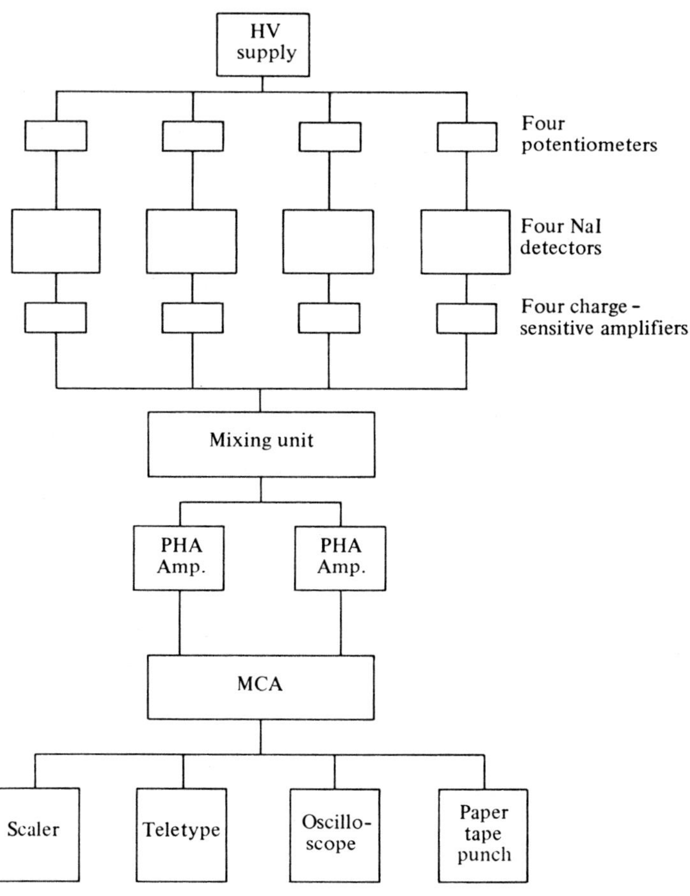

Fig. 8.5. Block diagram of associated electronic equipment for a whole-body counter.

(a) 3/8/77 ^{51}CR SPECTRUM C/100 SECS

00	000000	000815	000843	000896	000857	000835	000871	000893	000968	001006
01	001039	001088	001202	001286	001417	001522	001685	001902	001829	002035
02	002179	002465	002627	003091	003491	003728	004179	004174	004205	003934
03	003604	003330	002929	002649	002366	002219	002041	001905	001856	001817
04	001771	001697	001663	001643	001587	001617	001598	001595	001632	001596
05	001672	001742	001838	002004	002185	002603	003341	004381	006003	008223
06	010707	013992	017237	019482	021603	022084	021846	020061	017752	014811
07	011608	009037	006284	004444	002739	001842	001084	000649	000354	000195
08	000126	000097	000082	000056	000053	000050	000042	000051	000064	000056
09	000064	000034	000042	000055	000041	000043	000037	000048	000046	000054
10	000000									

(b)

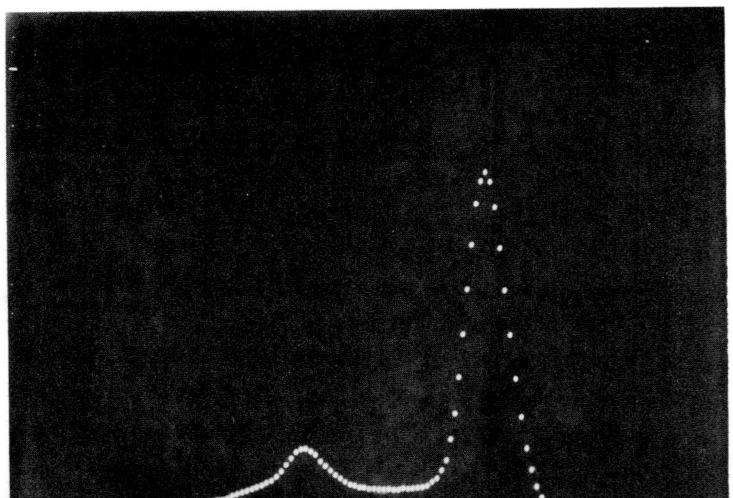

Fig. 8.6. Whole-body counter display from MCA in multiscaler mode, showing ^{51}Cr spectrum. (a) Teletype printout; (b) Polaroid photograph of oscilloscope; (c) curve drawn by computer from the data punched on to paper tape.

(c)

22084
0
10
20
30
40
50
60
70
80
90
100
STUDY NO.:1
,VIEW: 1
SPECTRUM?
CR51

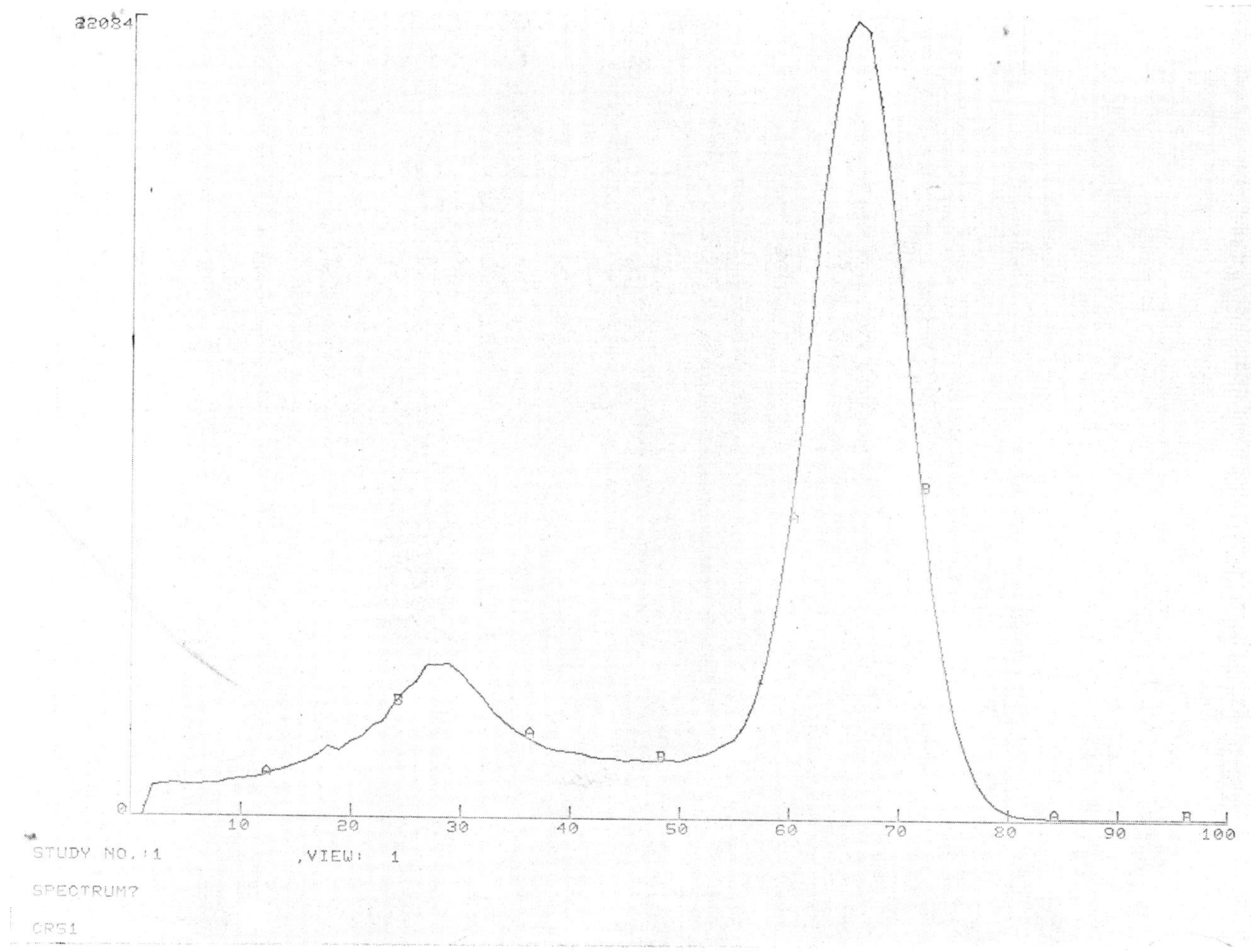

open collimator slit. The associated electronic equipment is shown schematically in Fig. 8.5. It comprises the HV supply to each of the four PM tubes, four charge-sensitive pre-amplifiers, one for each detector, and a mixing circuit which takes the output from each of the pre-amplifiers and provides at its output any required combination of these. The output from the mixing unit is fed via a single, or two, PHA and amplifier into a multichannel analyser (MCA), and this provides a very flexible system. An MCA may have 400 channels and can be programmed so that preselected groups of pulses are stored in each of the channels. The number of pulses collected in each channel can then be displayed as a frequency distribution on the oscilloscope, printed as a list of numbers by teletype, or punched out on to paper tape for subsequent computer processing. There are two main modes of operation usually known as multichannel and multiscaler.

Multichannel mode

In this mode the MCA is used to obtain the pulse-height distribution of the mixer circuit output; the MCA is set so that each of its 400 channels will accept pulses within a small discrete energy band. The couch on which the patient is positioned is made to move under the detectors so that the whole of the body is exposed in turn to the field of view. The total counts received from the body are thus obtained in the form of an energy spectrum (Fig. 8.6). This method provides no positional information and therefore the collimator slits may be adjusted to maximum width, which is obviously the most sensitive setting. The multichannel mode is useful for dual-nuclide studies since the spectra of the two nuclides can be selected from the overall spectrum, provided that their peaks are sufficiently far apart. For example, it is used for vitamin B12 absorption studies, when [^{58}Co] B12 may be used without intrinsic factor and [^{57}Co] B12 with intrinsic factor. This mode is also useful if it is required to compare the apparent distribution using the photopeak radiation emitted with that obtained using the Compton scattered radiation.

Multiscaler mode

In this mode the MCA is used to obtain the distribution of radioactivity along the length of the body, often referred to as a profile. The single PHA is used to select the channel width of pulses, usually the photopeak, to be transmitted to the MCA. The MCA is programmed so that the numbers of counts recorded in a preset time interval are sequentially stored in the 400 channels. As the patient moves under the collimator slits, each time interval corresponds to a discrete movement of the couch and a small transverse section of the body is centred in turn under the detectors. By reducing the collimation to a narrow slit, good spatial resolution can be achieved and the resultant MCA distribution represents a profile of the distribution within the body (Fig. 8.7). This mode is particularly useful for detection of metastases in thyroid carcinoma. A fairly large tracer dose (1 mCi or 37 MBq) of ^{131}I is given to the patient, and when the blood level has cleared at 3 or 4 days a profile distribution is obtained (Fig. 8.7). A peak which persists for several days is evidence of ^{131}I uptake, which can then be further investigated by two-dimensional imaging.

If the output of the mixer circuit is fed into two PHAs dual-nuclide studies can be carried out and profiles obtained simultaneously for two nuclides.

Imaging systems

Rectilinear scanners and gamma cameras as used in static imaging have been described in Chapter 7. Dynamic studies in the sense of serial images carried out daily, or even hourly, are possible with rectilinear scanners and are often useful. The advent of single-crystal and multi-crystal gamma cameras, however, opened up the

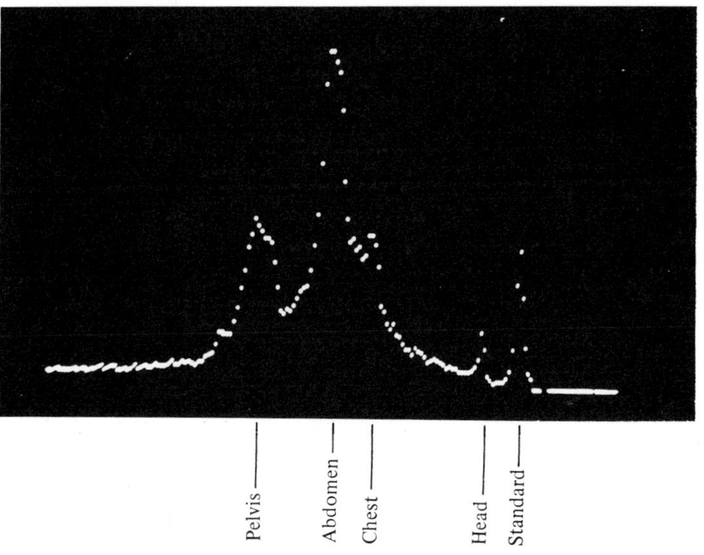

Fig. 8.7. Whole-body counter display from MCA in multichannel mode, showing profile of patient with carcinoma of the thyroid.

possibility of rapid dynamic studies capable of demonstrating changes in distribution taking place in time intervals as short as tenths of a second. There are applications in blood-flow measurements and in cardiology as well as renography. Such studies are possible because the gamma camera can view the whole field of view at the same time; they are dependent on data collection facilities which are essential for quantitative results, and also on data processing facilities. It is the development of these latter devices which has given great impetus to dynamic imaging techniques. Chapter 9 gives a brief account of the computer equipment and processing.

The gamma camera is set up in precisely the same manner for dynamic studies as for static studies, except that the patient is positioned before the injection of radioactive material. The injection is given as a rapid bolus and counts are recorded from the time of injection. Renographic studies are done in much the same way as probe renography, but accurate positioning is not necessary because the regions of interest, that is the kidney or any particular part of the kidney, can be selected retrospectively for quantitative analysis. Blood-flow studies, for example cerebral blood flow, may be carried out using a radiopharmaceutical which remains in the vascular system, e.g. [^{99m}Tc] HSA. The gamma camera is positioned over the vertex of the head and counts are recorded during the first passage of the radioactive material through the head. A single probe may be positioned over the aortic root to provide the input curve to the cerebral circulation. The method of analysis of the curves is described later.

Equilibrium studies

Phelps (Phelps, Hoffman & Kuhl, 1977) has viewed the dynamic process as a summation or accumulation of data and has used sophisticated techniques with positron emitters to investigate regional cerebral perfusion and metabolism. Computerised emission tomography (annihilation coincidence detection) was carried out 4 to 5 minutes after the intravenous injection of $^{13}NH_3$. Experiments on monkeys after carotid injection had shown that about 50% of the $^{13}NH_3$ is extracted in the first circulation and retained by the cerebral tissues, with a washout half-time of about 45 minutes. Less than 2% is recirculated, the remainder being exhaled. The distribution of activity within the tomographic sections therefore represents the blood perfusion distribution, which is dependent on capillary distribution, and diffusion of ammonia across the blood–brain barrier. By repeating the tomography after inhalation of ^{11}CO, which labelled the blood with [^{11}CO]haemoglobin, the distribution of the blood vessels was obtained. The combined study may provide a means of distinguishing between large and small vessel involvement in pathological changes. $^{13}NH_3$ and ^{11}CO have also been used by the above author for myocardial imaging. Unfortunately the use of these techniques is restricted since they require not only a complex ECAT machine but also an on-site cyclotron to provide the short-lived positron emitters.

Data analysis

The power of dynamic studies is that the data can be analysed to provide information about physiological processes such as flow rate, exchange rate, etc. A common approach is to put forward a physical or mathematical model which is thought to simulate the behaviour of the system under investigation, and the experimental data are fed into this model in order to obtain the required result. A detailed discussion of analytical methods is outside the scope of this book and the reader is referred to a comprehensive survey by Sheppard (1962). The functions of interest are rate of uptake, diffusion, transport, metabolism and excretion, and blood flow. It is often not possible to isolate any one of these functions for measurement, the data which can be obtained are the input, accumulation and removal of radioactivity from an organ and from the blood.

Deconvolution

The shape of the output (OP) curve from any system will depend on the shape of the input (IP) curve and also on the response of the system. The latter may provide valuable information regarding its function, and may be described in terms of the time it takes for the material to be transported through the system, normally known as transit time, (t). There is usually a distribution of transit times $h(t)$ which may be represented by a curve of $h(t)$ against time. In renography the [^{131}I]hippuran in the arterial supply to the glomerulus is transported through the nephrons to the pelvi-ureteric junction, and the transit time spectrum is of interest.

The response of a system may be demonstrated by introducing a 'spike' injection at the input and observing the output from the system, which will give the transit time spectrum. Alternatively, the retention in the system may be observed and the negative differential of the retention function will yield the transit time spectrum. A 'spike' injection is one in which all the radioactivity is injected instantaneously; in practice it is not always possible to introduce a spike input, and the output curve is a convolution of the input curve and the response function. This is expressed mathematically:

$$\mathrm{OP} = \mathrm{IP} * h(t) \tag{8.5}$$

If the input curve and output or retention curve can be obtained the techniques of deconvolution can be applied to obtain the transit time spectrum.

The concept of convolution can be explained by a simple illustration (Fig. 8.8). In (*a*) the system has a single transit time T shown in (*a*1), the input is a spike occurring at $t = 0$ (*a*2), the retention is given in (*a*3) which shows all the radioactivity entering the system at $t = 0$, being retained for a period of time equal

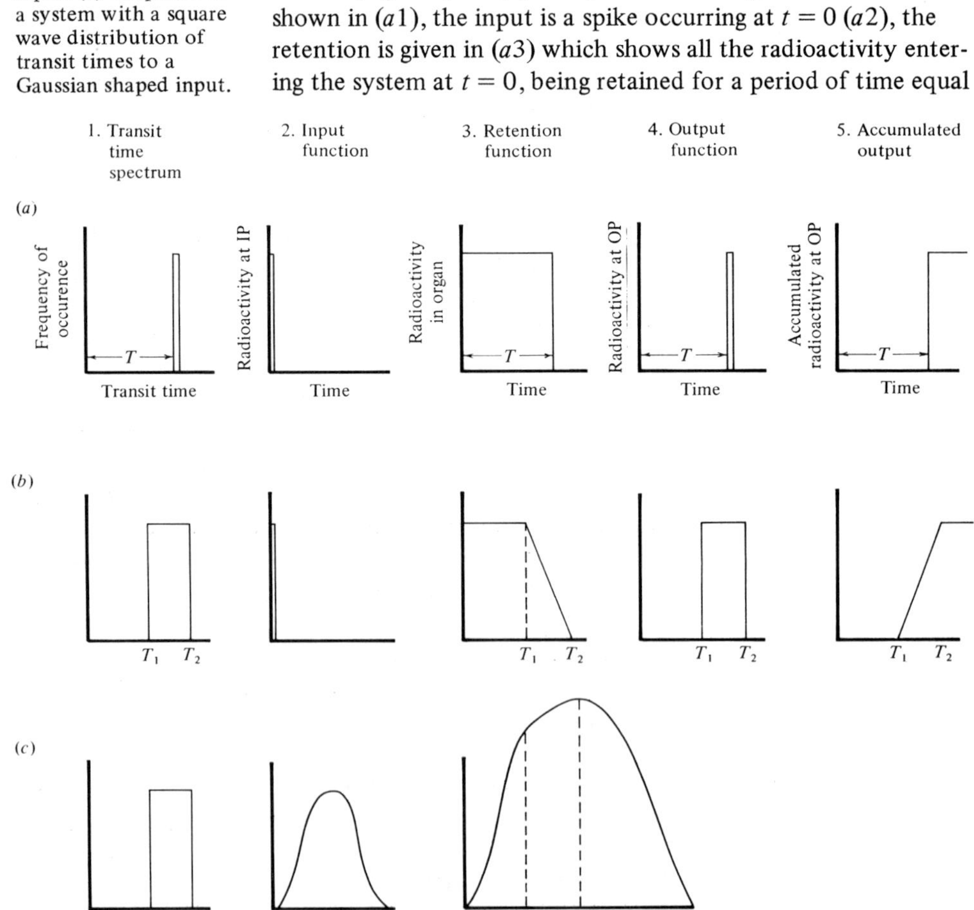

Fig. 8.8. Diagrammatic representation of convolution. (*a*) Response of system with single transit time to a spike input. (*b*) Response of system with a square wave distribution of transit times to a spike input. (*c*) Response of a system with a square wave distribution of transit times to a Gaussian shaped input.

to the transit time T and then all leaving the system when t equals T. The output curve (a4) shows all the radioactivity reaching the output at the same time when $t = T$; (a5) gives the accumulated output. Fig. 8.8(b) shows the response of a system with a square wave distribution of transit times ranging from T_1 to T_2 (b1), to a spike input (b2). The retention curve (b3) shows all the radioactivity entering the system at $t = 0$, remaining in the system until $t = T_1$, after which time equal amounts will leave per unit time up to $t = T_2$, so that the retention falls linearly to zero at $t = T_2$. The output curve (b4) is again the same as the transit time distribution. It should be noted that the transit time distribution is the negative differential of the retention curve. Fig. 8.8(c) shows the response of a system with a square wave distribution of transit times to an input with a Gaussian distribution. The retention curve (c3) shows the radioactivity beginning to enter the system at $t = 0$, following the shape of the integrated input curve up to the time when $t = T$, then flattening off and decreasing until it reaches zero at a time $t = T_2 + T_3$.

Application to renography

In renography the arterial input function to the kidney can be obtained from the blood clearance curve. The curve of total kidney content if there were no excretion can be obtained by fitting the integral of the blood clearance curve to the initial part of the renogram, that is the period before any radioactivity leaves the kidney. The output curve can then be obtained by subtracting the input curve from the total. Deconvolution techniques can be applied; deconvoluting the corrected total renogram with the blood curve yields the retention function which on differentiation gives the transit time spectrum. This is illustrated in Fig. 9.5. Deconvoluting the output curve with the integral of the blood curve gives the transit time spectrum directly.

Application to measurement of blood flow

The concept of transit times can also be used to measure blood flow. The mean transit time of radioactive label through a system is related to the mean blood flow rate and the volume of distribution by the following equation (Zierler, 1962):

$$F = V/\bar{t} \tag{8.6}$$

where F = flow rate in ml per second
V = volume of distribution of the tracer in ml
$\bar{t}$ = mean transit time in seconds

If V and $\bar{t}$ can be measured, then F can be calculated. Continuous measurement of the radioactivity in the region of interest, after a bolus injection, yields an activity–time curve of the type shown in Fig. 8.8(c3). If the input curve approximates to a spike then the mean transit time is approximately equal to the abscissal value of the centroid of the activity–time curve, given by the equation

$$\bar{t} = \frac{\int t\, A(t)\, \mathrm{d}t}{\int A(t)\, \mathrm{d}t} \tag{8.7}$$

A more accurate value is obtained by deconvoluting the first circulation curve with the input curve. The latter is obtained from the counts recorded by the detector over the aortic root. The

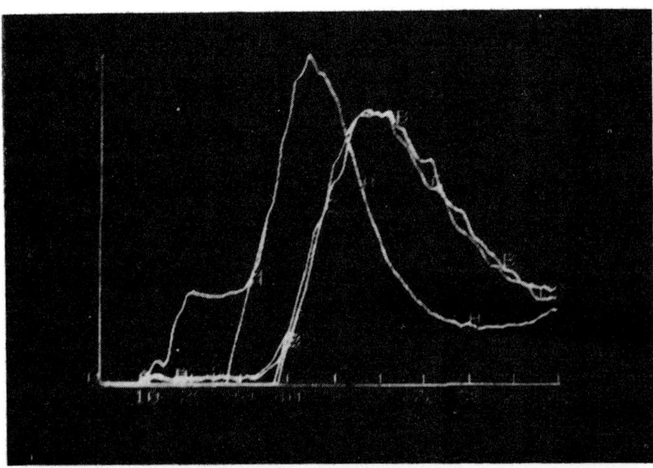

(a)

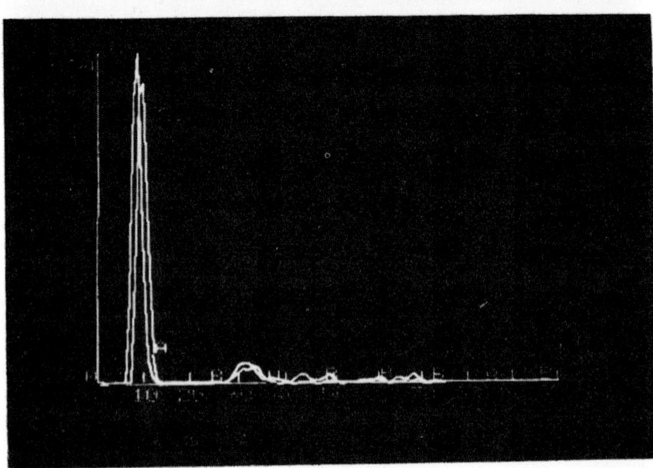

(b)

Fig. 8.9. (a) Activity–time curves after a bolus injection, with detectors over the aortic root, and the two carotid arteries. (b) Transit time spectra for the two arteries obtained by deconvolution of the curves in (a).

result of deconvolution is the retention function curve, which when differentiated gives the transit time spectra. A value for V, the blood volume of the region under study, is obtained by taking a measurement at equilibrium which can be calibrated in terms of the concentration in a blood sample taken at the time of that measurement. It should be noted that certain assumptions are implicit in the above. These are: that the system is linear, that the response of the system is constant during the period of study, and that the tracer is uniformly mixed at the input point of observation. Also, for equation 8.6 to be valid, complete mixing of tracer between input and output is assumed. Fig. 8.9(*a*) shows activity–time curves after a bolus injection with detectors over the aortic root (IP) and over the two carotid arteries (OP). Fig. 8.9(*b*) shows the transit time spectra for the two arteries, obtained by deconvolution of the above curves; it demonstrates single transit times in each artery.

References

Phelps, M.E., Hoffman, E.J. & Kuhl, D.E. (1977). Physiologic tomography (PT) a new approach to in vivo measure of metabolism and physiologic function. In *Medical Radionuclide Imaging*, vol. 1, pp. 233–51. Vienna: International Atomic Energy Agency.

Phelps, M.E. (1977). What is the purpose of emission computed tomography in nuclear medicine. *J. Nucl. Med.* **18**, 399–402.

Sheppard, C.W. (1962). *Basic Principles of the Tracer Method*, New York: Wiley.

Zierler, K.L. (1962). Theoretical basis of indicator-dilution methods for measuring flow and volume. *Circ. Res.* **10**, 393–407.

9. Data collection and processing

Introduction

It was pointed out in the last chapter that fast dynamic studies are dependent on the availability of data collection and data processing facilities. This chapter is concerned with these facilities as applied to gamma cameras. A computer is required to collect the data, and handle them in the form of a matrix to produce one single or many sequential images, which can be displayed. From sequential images the computer is required to produce activity–time curves for any region of interest. A so-called interactive system is essential, in order that the operator may alter conditions so that the image is displayed to greatest advantage.

Hardware

The actual equipment is referred to as the hardware of the system. Fig. 9.1(*a*) shows a block diagram of the essential features, which are an input, analogue-to-digital converters (ADC), an input–

Fig. 9.1. (*a*) Block diagram of essential features of a data processing system. (*b*) Block diagram of a typical system.

(*a*)

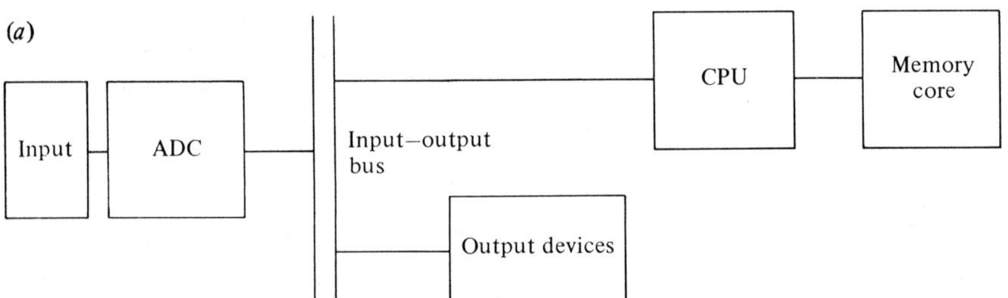

(*b*)

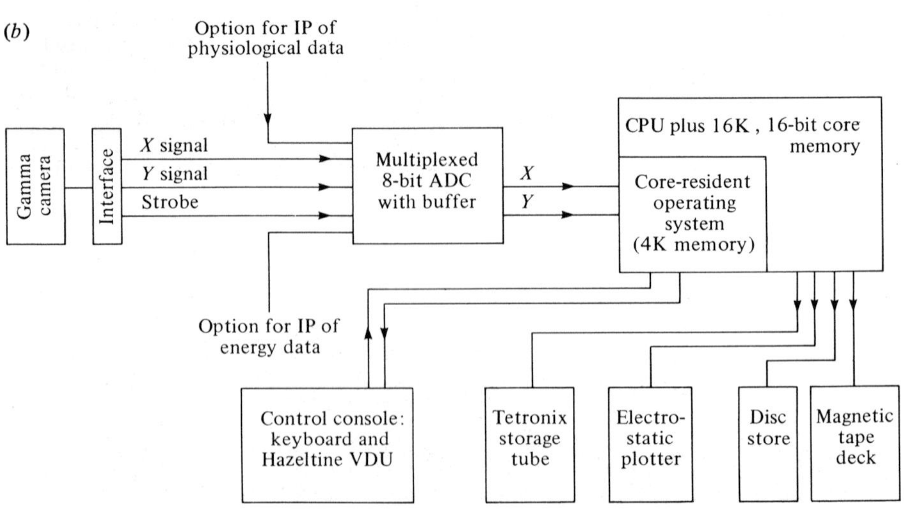

output bus or controller, a central processing unit (CPU), memory store or core and output devices. Fig. 9.1(*b*) shows a block diagram of a typical system comprising: a gamma camera interface (to obtain the gamma camera output data in a form compatible with the computer input), ADC with buffer, a control console with a visual display unit (VDU) and keyboard which acts as an interactive system, and a CPU with a 4K core-resident operating system, plus 16K core memory. (In computer language 1K equals 1024 or 2^{10} storage locations.) There are several output devices: disc unit and magnetic tape unit for storage of data; tetronix storage tube or TV monitor for displaying images or curves; and there may also be an electrostatic plotter to produce permanent hard copies. A photograph of this system is shown in Fig. 9.2.

Software

Computer programs are instructions, written in a computer language such as Fortran, which tell the computer what to do with the data fed into it. They are referred to as software. Software packages are usually commercially available for corrections of field non-uniformity, for background subtraction, contrast

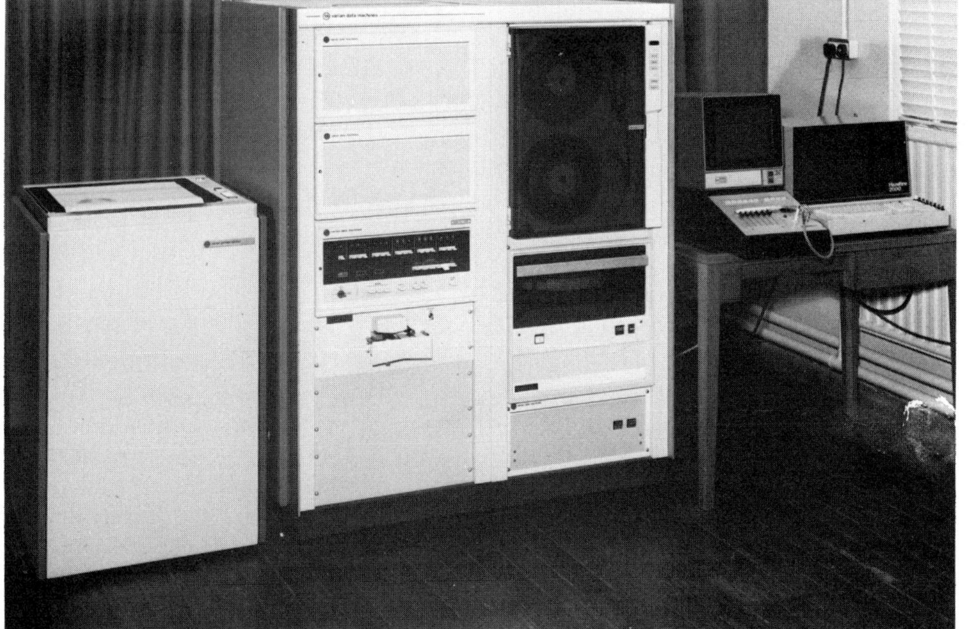

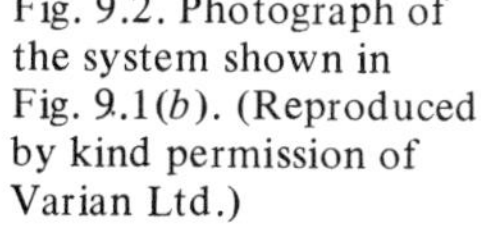

Fig. 9.2. Photograph of the system shown in Fig. 9.1(*b*). (Reproduced by kind permission of Varian Ltd.)

enhancement, and contour plotting. By further program development more sophisticated analysis can be achieved.

Data collection

It was shown (p. 106) that the gamma camera provides three output pulses for each photon detected in the crystal; the X and Y pulses are proportional to the coordinates of the point in the crystal where the scintillation is produced, and the Z pulse is proportional to the amplitude of the output pulse due to that scintillation. ADCs change these analogue signals to digital ones. There are two ways of collecting data: in the form of a matrix, or as a list. These will be denoted by incremental or sequential mode, respectively.

Incremental mode

In this mode the data are formed into matrices as they are collected. A matrix is a series of numerical values arranged in rows and columns. In this context, each pulse is assigned to a position, or element, in the matrix which corresponds to its X and Y coordinates. The numerical value given to any element of the matrix is equal to the number of pulses assigned to that element during the time of data collection, often referred to as a frame. The number of elements which can be handled in this mode is limited by the computer memory store. For example, a 64 × 64 matrix contains 4096 (i.e. 4K) elements, and a 128 × 128 matrix contains 16 384 (i.e. 16K), so that while a 4K memory store will handle the former it will not handle the latter. The spatial resolution of the image is limited by the number of elements in the matrix; with a camera having a field of view of 25 cm diameter the elements in a 64 × 64 matrix will be of size 25 cm divided by 64, that is 4 mm square.

For any investigation on a patient, the data may be collected for the whole period in one frame; for example, a static image of a brain is obtained by collecting data over the 4 or 5 minutes it takes to produce a direct photographic picture. Alternatively, the collection of data may be divided up into several frames each of short duration, for example one-tenth of a second or one second. Each frame when complete is transferred to disc storage, to allow collection of the next frame. The frames can subsequently be retrieved from the disc store, and since each is formed as a matrix it is immediately available for display on the storage oscilloscope. The raw data are the same as the data which produce the direct photodisplay, but the image is quantised into elements. This difference is evident in some displays but in others the data is 'dequantised' before display to avoid the chequerboard effect.

Sequential mode

The X and Y coordinates of each pulse are recorded sequentially as they occur, and also the pulse-height energy Z if required. Time marks are made at specified intervals such as 1 millisecond. The precision with which the coordinates are recorded will be of the order of 1 mm, corresponding to one element in a 256 × 256 matrix with a 25 cm field-of-view camera. It is evident that because there are more data for each pulse, much greater storage space is required for sequential mode acquisition than for incremental mode; also it may be count-rate limited, that is unable to handle such high count-rates as the incremental mode. For example, for incremental mode the maximum input rate may be 70 000 counts per second with no practical limit to the total number of counts, whereas for sequential mode the maximum input rate may be 36 000 counts per second with the total number of counts limited by disc storage space, typically to 2 000 000. On the other hand, in incremental mode the spatial resolution is limited, often to 4 mm. In general, incremental acquisition is used for routine work, and sequential acquisition for studies where high spatial resolution is required. The latter has the advantage that frames can be selected retrospectively.

Initial data processing

The data collected in list mode can be put into matrix form, and then be handled in the same way as incremental mode data. Images may be formed from the raw data, or after the operations of background subtraction, smoothing and filtration have been carried out. For routine work there will usually be a standard protocol which the computer will follow, and then display the type of image selected.

Display of images

There are generally four different forms of display: grey scale, colour, contours and isometric projection. These may be produced on a storage oscilloscope or TV screen, or as a hard copy. The grey scale is probably the most common; it is produced by using analogue signals, proportional to the number of pulses in each matrix element, to vary the brightness in each element or the number of dots printed in each element. The quantised nature of display which results from the above can be reduced by interpolating the scales of grey. In colour display the analogue signals are divided into a definite number of colours, with colour changes at somewhat arbitrary levels (but these can easily be varied). Colour has the advantage that it makes it very easy to recognise discrete levels of activity. In contour display, isocount curves are plotted at levels which may vary almost continuously from zero up to the maximum count, thus providing a quantitative assessment of the percentage difference of count-rate in an abnormality from that in its surroundings. The isometric display provides a three-dimensional view of the matrix.

Fig. 9.3 shows the static right lateral image of a brain displayed in five ways: (*a*) is the direct gamma camera image photographed on transparent film from the camera oscilloscope; (*b*) is a computer 64 × 64 matrix display in shades of grey; (*c*) is an interpolated display with a 128 × 128 matrix; (*d*) is as (*c*) with a 25% background subtraction and contrast enhancement; and (*e*) is a contour plot.

The great advantage of computer display in a static study, compared with the direct photographic display routinely used, is that it provides an interactive means of varying background and contrast. It can also provide quantitative information such as the rate of counts in a suspect area to those in a normal area.

Regions of interest and dynamic curves

In a dynamic study it is possible to display the matrices of sequential frames on the storage oscilloscope and these may give a qualitative idea of function. But the data contain quantitative information regarding the variation of activity with time in each element of the matrix, and can be used to plot an activity–time curve for any region of interest (ROI). For example, in a renography study, a good image (obtained by summing all frames recorded during the study) is displayed as above on the oscilloscope, and then two ROIs are formed to outline the two kidneys. This may be done by using contours or by manually operating a light bug across the oscilloscope. On selection of the appropriate program the computer will integrate the data over each ROI and plot an activity–time curve for each kidney. Fig. 9.4(*a*) shows the computer display of two kidneys, with both kidneys and renal pelves outlined as ROIs, and (*b*) and (*c*) show the dynamic curves for right and left kidneys respectively, each giving the curve for the whole kidney, the renal pelvis and the whole kidney minus the pelvis.

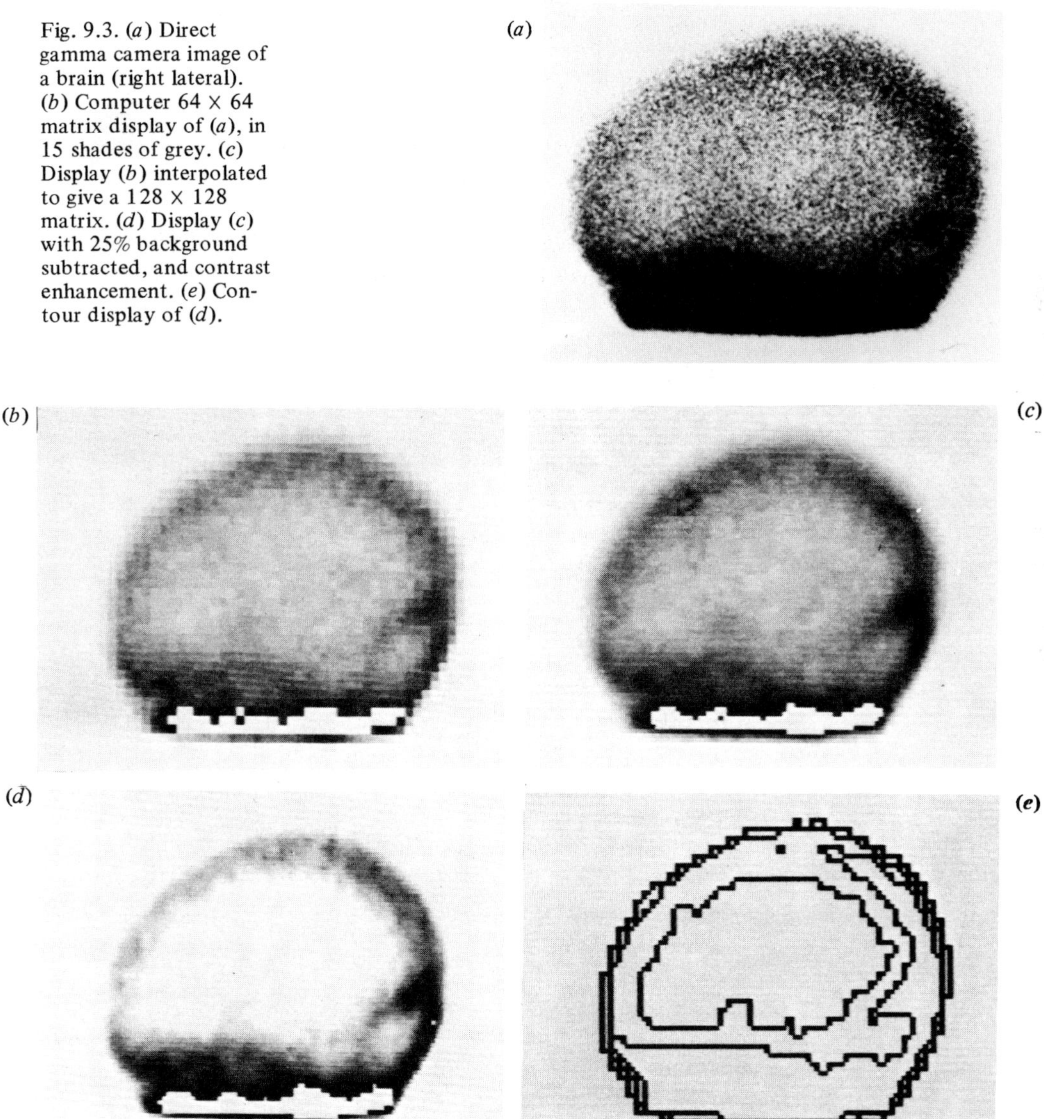

Fig. 9.3. (*a*) Direct gamma camera image of a brain (right lateral). (*b*) Computer 64 × 64 matrix display of (*a*), in 15 shades of grey. (*c*) Display (*b*) interpolated to give a 128 × 128 matrix. (*d*) Display (*c*) with 25% background subtracted, and contrast enhancement. (*e*) Contour display of (*d*).

(*a*)

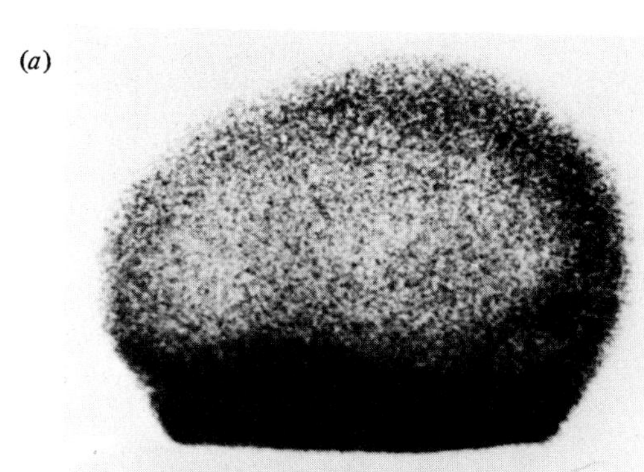

(*b*)

(*c*)

(*d*)

(*e*)

(a)

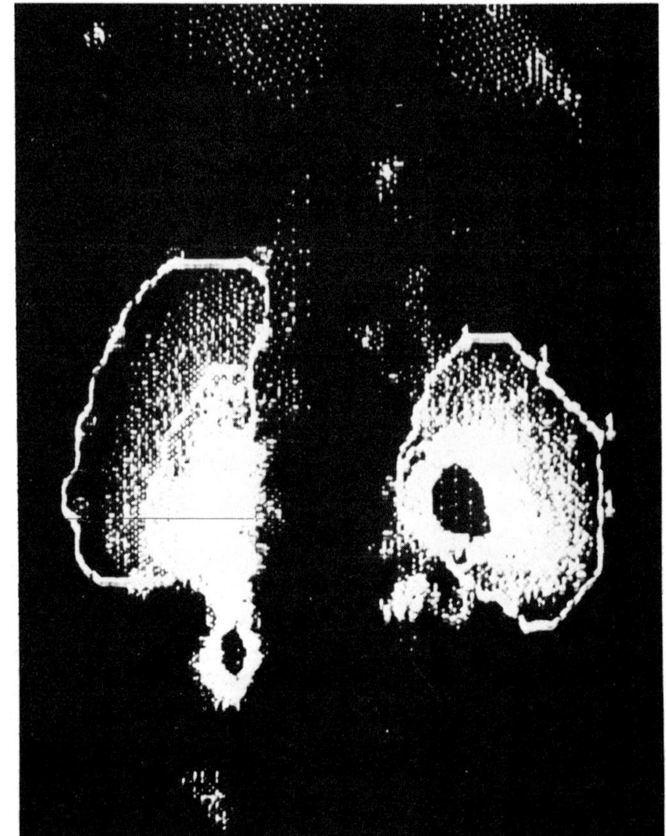

Fig. 9.4. (a) Computer 64 × 64 matrix display of the two kidneys, with four ROIs defined: left kidney and renal pelvis, right kidney and renal pelvis. (b) and (c) Dynamic curves for the right and left kidneys respectively: *A* whole kidney; *B* renal pelvis; *C* whole kidney plus pelvis.

(b)

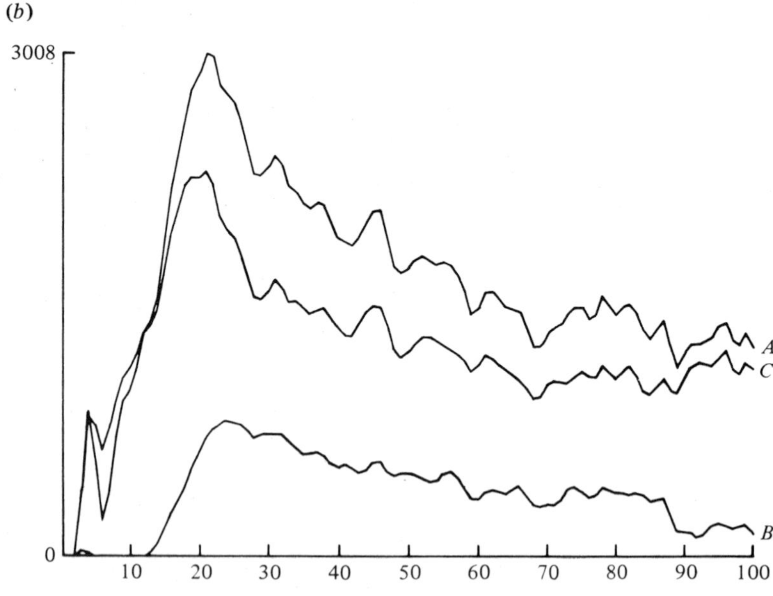

More sophisticated data

Deconvolution

Computer technology can be used to apply the deconvolution techniques referred to in Chapter 8. Fig. 9.5 shows the results of a dynamic renal study: (*a*) shows the right kidney curve and the sub-clavicular curve, (*b*) the retention function curve obtained by deconvoluting the above two curves, and (*c*) the transit time spectrum obtained by differentiating (*b*).

Functional imaging

The normal routine display of images shows the mean distribution of radioactivity over the period of collection. Other parameters which reflect the function of an organ may provide useful additional information if their distribution is similarly displayed. For example, in a cerebral blood flow study, functional images showing the distribution of the activity integrated over the first circulation, and the mean time (as obtained from the centroid of the activity–time curve) (Fig. 9.6*a* and *b*) reflect the blood flow, whereas the conventional image of equilibrium distribution (Fig. 9.6*c*) reflects blood volume.

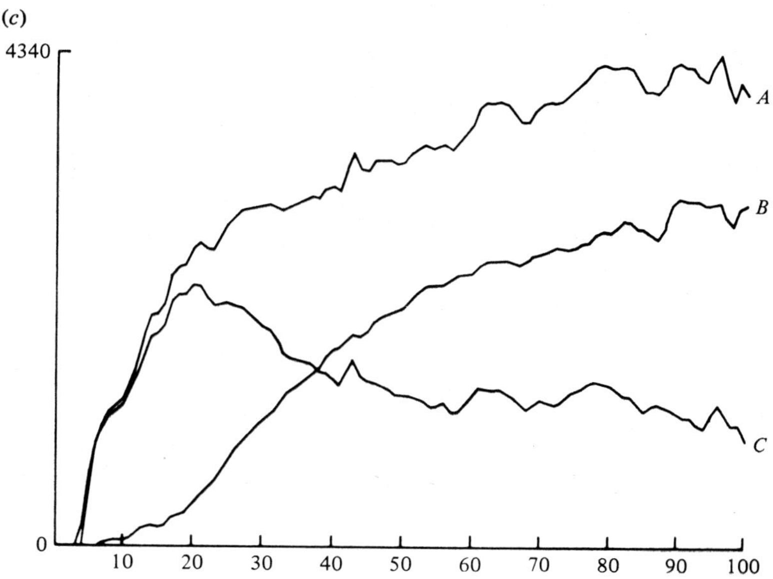

Fig. 9.5. (*a*) Dynamic curves for right kidney (upper line) and subclavicular region (lower line). (*b*) Retention function curve obtained from two curves shown in (*a*). (*c*) Transit time spectrum obtained by differentiation of (*b*).

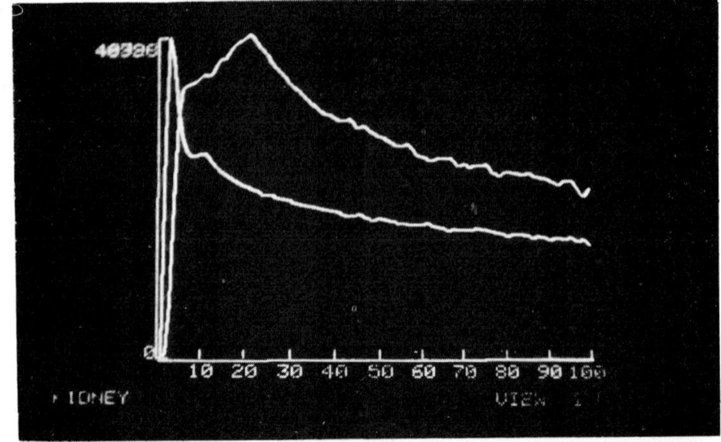

(*a*)

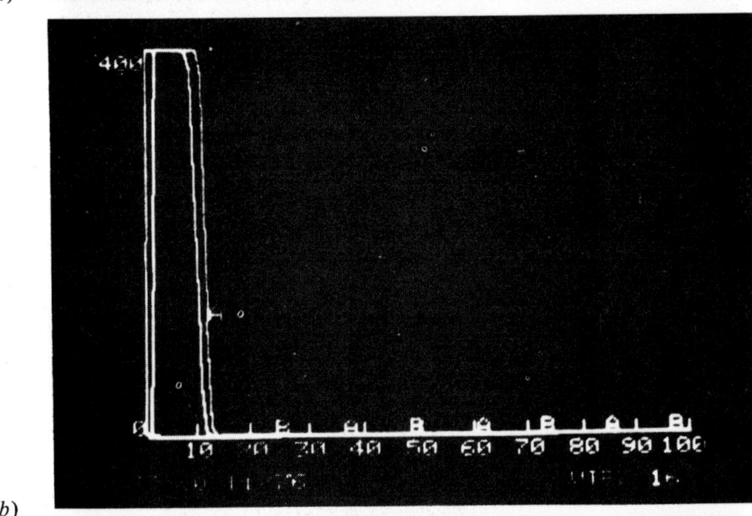

(*b*)

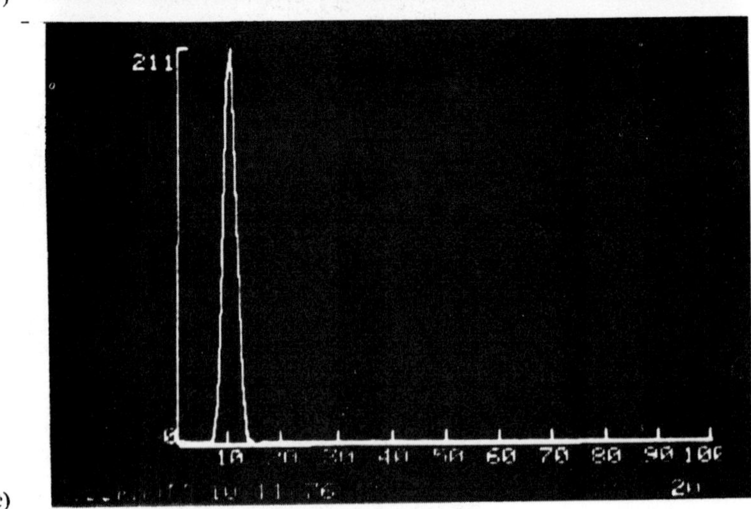

(*c*)

Fig. 9.6. Functional imaging in cerebral blood flow. (*a*) Activity integrated over the time of the first circulation; (*b*) mean time; (*c*) equilibrium distribution.

(*a*)

(*b*)

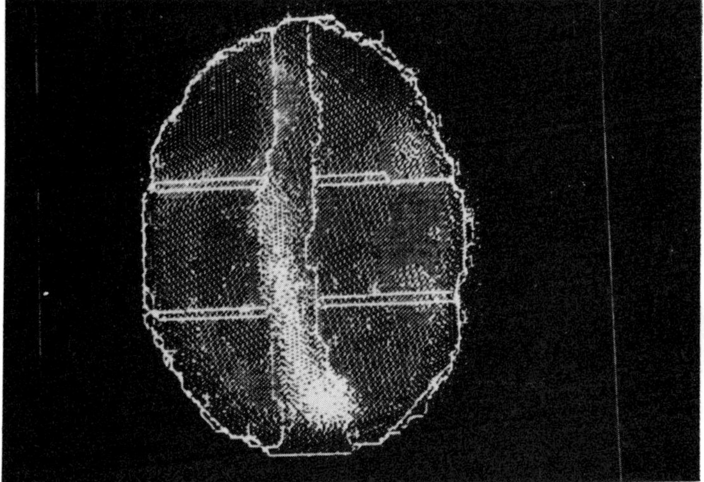

(*c*)

Comparison with normal image

A great deal of work has been done, particularly related to static brain imaging, on detecting abnormalities by computer. Three lines of approach have been used: many workers have obtained the 'normal' images from a series of clinically proven normals, and used subtraction techniques to display any abnormality (Dowsett & Perry, 1970; Cormack & McAlister, 1972); Brown, Budd & Britton (1975) have compared a suspected abnormal area with its surroundings; and Barber (1976) has used the method of principal components.

Data processing for multi-crystal camera

Because, as described in Chapter 7, in a multi-crystal camera the system acts as a number of individual crystals and therefore the detection and positioning of events are independent, it can operate at higher count-rates than a single-crystal camera without saturating the detectors or introducing non-correctable positioning distortions. Typically it can operate at about 2.3×10^5 counts per second, compared with a maximum of about 0.5×10^5 counts per second for the single-crystal camera. This higher count-rate capability is an important feature in dynamic studies, where short sampling times of 0.01 to 0.05 seconds are essential and reasonable statistics can only be obtained at high count-rates. On the other hand, short sampling times prohibit the use of the 16-position mode, so that spatial resolution is limited by the crystal-to-crystal spacing; this is overcome by using temporal resolution.

An essential feature of the data handling system is a fast solid-state buffer containing 294 memory locations, one for each crystal, which is used to store temporarily all events during the accumulation period. The entire contents of the buffer memory are transferred to the computer core every second during a static measurement, and after every accumulation interval during a dynamic study. The data are then transferred to disc store for future retrieval, or magnetic tape for permanent storage. Corrections for non-uniformity of crystal response, for background, and for dead-time losses at high count-rates can be carried out automatically.

The matrix display uses either a scale of 16 grey shades or 16 separate colours each corresponding to 6.25% increments in counts. As with the single-crystal gamma camera it is possible to select ROIs and plot dynamic curves. Dynamic studies can also be displayed as serial images or in ciné mode, which is particularly instructive in cardiac studies.

Fig. 9.7. (*a*) Left ventricle outline at end-diastole. (*b*) Left ventricle outline at end-systole. (*c*) Subtraction of (*b*) from (*a*), demonstrating the movement of the left ventricular wall. (Photographs reproduced by courtesy of Baird-Atomic Ltd.)

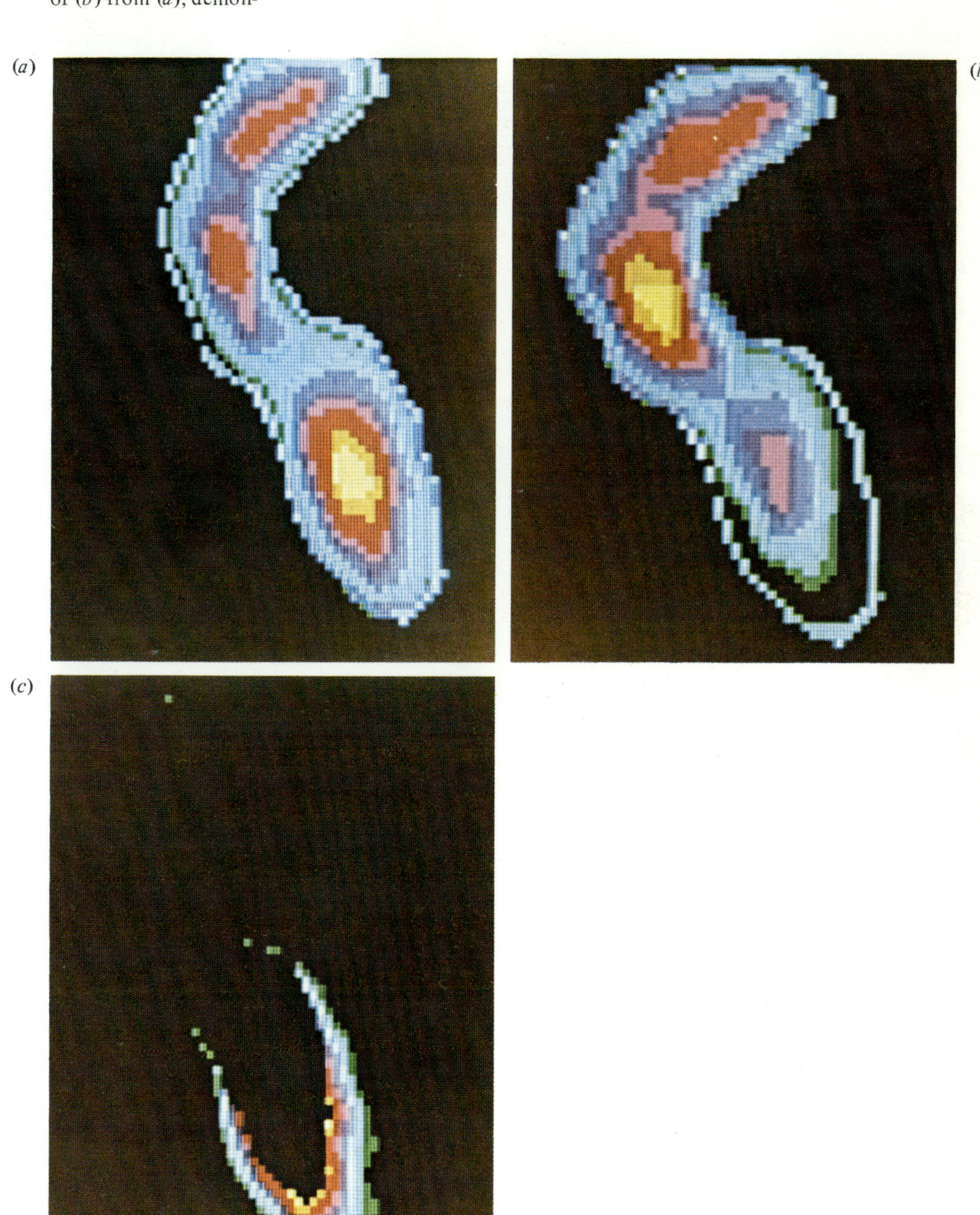

One important application of this system lies in quantitative measurements of the cardiac cycle. After a bolus injection of ^{99m}Tc, data are collected over a period of 50 seconds, which covers the first passage through the central circulatory system. The edges of the heart chambers can be clearly delineated in end-diastole and end-systole (Fig. 9.7*a* and *b*) by summing each statistically significant frame of each part of the cycle. For example, the 100 millisecond frame at end-diastole will occur perhaps four times during the first passage, and by using a gating system based on either an electrocardiograph or a time cycle, the sum of these four can be obtained, and will provide better statistics for the end-diastole image. Alternatively, when equilibrium distribution of radioactivity has been reached, a larger number of cycles can be summated, using gating to identify each part of the cardiac cycle. By subtracting the end-systole image from the end-diastole image, the range of the chamber wall movement can be displayed and measured (Fig. 9.7*c*).

References

Barber, D.C. (1976). Digital computer processing of brain scans using principal components. *Phys. Med. Biol.* **21**, 792–803.

Brown, N.J.G., Budd, T. & Britton, K.E. (1975). On the transmission of quantitative difference information via an interactive computer system to the clinical interpreter. In *Information Processing in Scintigraphy*, ed. C. Raynaud & A. Todd-Pokropek, pp. 377–89. Orsay: Commisariat à l'Energie Atomique.

Cormack, J. & McAlister, J. (1972). Digital techniques and displays in brain scanning. *Neuroradiol.* **4**, 171–8.

Dowsett, D.J. & Perry, B.J. (1970). A comparative statistical analysis of brain scans using a digital computer. *B. J. Radiol.* **43**, 617–28.

10. Fundamental theory

A brief introduction to the theory of radioactivity was given in Chapter 2; in this chapter it is considered in more detail.

Fundamental particles and atomic structure

Radioactivity is a phenomenon associated with the nucleus of the atom. In order to understand it, it is necessary to know something about the structure of the atom, and the periodic classification of the elements. All matter is made up from approximately 100 elements, and the atom is the structural unit of an element.

There are three fundamental particles associated with the atom – the proton, the neutron and the electron (Table 10.1). The proton and neutron are relatively heavy particles, with mass approximately one atomic mass unit ($1\ m_u = 1.66 \times 10^{-24}$ g); the proton bears one fundamental unit of charge (1.60×10^{-19} C) and the neutron is electrically neutral. The electron is a very light particle, with mass $0.00055 m_u$, and one fundamental unit of negative charge.

Another particle which is encountered in radioactivity is the positron, with mass the same as that of the electron but with one fundamental unit of positive charge. There are also uncharged particles of very small mass, known as neutrinos, but they are virtually undetectable and need not be considered here.

The atom may be considered as consisting of a central nucleus and orbital electrons. The nucleus is composed of the heavy particles: protons and neutrons. The number of protons in the nucleus determines the positive charge on the nucleus and is called the atomic number (Z). It denotes the place occupied by the element in the Periodic Table. The number of protons plus neutrons determines the weight of the atom and is called the mass number (A). Normally the atom is electrically neutral so that the number of electrons is equal to the number of protons. Chemical reactions involve only interaction between electrons, and the chemical properties of an atom are therefore determined by the number of electrons, that is they are characterised by the atomic number.

Table 10.1 *Fundamental particles*

		Mass (m_u)	Charge (C)
Proton	In nucleus	1.00727	$+1.602 \times 10^{-19}$
Neutron	In nucleus	1.00866	None
Electron	Outside nucleus	0.00055	-1.602×10^{-19}

An element is matter consisting of atoms having the same atomic number, that is of atoms having identical chemical properties. The number of neutrons in the atom of an element may vary, and therefore its mass number may vary. Let us consider, for example, hydrogen, which is the first element in the periodic table. Naturally occurring hydrogen has two types of atom: ${}^{1}_{1}H$ which comprises 99.984% of the total atoms and has one proton in its nucleus (i.e. its atomic number is 1 and its mass number is also 1), and ${}^{2}_{1}H$ which comprises 0.0155% of the total atoms and has one proton and one neutron in its nucleus (i.e. its atomic number is 1 and its mass number is 2). ${}^{2}_{1}H$ is also known as deuterium or 'heavy hydrogen' and is used to make 'heavy water'. The nucleus of its atom is referred to as a deuteron. Naturally occurring oxygen (atomic number 8) has three types of atom, each with 8 protons but with 8, 9 and 10 neutrons respectively, i.e. ${}^{16}_{8}O$, ${}^{17}_{8}O$ and ${}^{18}_{8}O$. The atomic weight of an element is dependent on the relative abundance of the isotopes and their mass numbers.

A nuclide is defined as a species of atom with a certain atomic number, mass number and nuclear energy state. Isotopes are nuclides having the same atomic number but with different mass numbers. Thus ${}^{1}H$ and ${}^{2}H$ are nuclides which are both isotopes of hydrogen. In common usage the term isotope is often used in place of the term nuclide; throughout this book the words isotope and nuclide are used in correct terminology, as defined above. The composition of a nuclide can be denoted (as above) by the atomic number as a subscript to the symbol for the element and the mass number as a superscript, e.g. ${}^{16}_{8}O$. However, since the symbol of the element is in itself characteristic of the atomic number, the subscript is usually omitted, e.g. ${}^{16}O$.

Radioactivity

The phenomenon of radioactivity, or radioactive decay, is the spontaneous disintegration of atomic nuclei; it occurs when the nucleus of a nuclide is unstable. In stable nuclides the relative number of protons and neutrons lies between quite close limits. When these limits are exceeded, i.e. when there is an excess or shortage of neutrons, the nucleus becomes unstable and tends to try to return to a stable configuration with the emission of radiation. For each nuclide its radioactive decay is characterised by the primary mode of decay and the energy released, the associated γ-radiation and its energy, and the decay (disintegration) constant. As a result of the spontaneous disintegration of the atomic nucleus, its atomic number is altered, that is transmutation of the element has taken place, a phenomenon which was sought by the alchemists in days gone by. Details of radioactive decay schemes may be found in the *Table of Isotopes* prepared by Lederer, Hollander & Perlman (1967), *The Radiochemical Manual* (Wilson, 1966), and Dillman & Von der Lage (1975).

Primary modes of decay

There are four main primary processes: alpha-emission, beta-emission, positron-emission and electron capture.

Alpha-emission. This is a process whereby the nucleus emits alpha-particles (α-particles), as in the well-known case of radium-226. The α-particles are the nuclei of stable helium atoms, ^4He, and consist of two protons and two neutrons, that is have a mass number of 4 and two positive units of charge. For reasons discussed later, this type of radiation is of little use in medical diagnostic work, and will not be considered further.

Beta-emission. This is a primary radioactive decay process in which, as the name implies, a beta-particle (β-particle) is emitted. A beta-particle is an electron; the term β-particle was used to describe the radiation before its nature was understood. This type of decay usually occurs in radioactive nuclides produced in a nuclear reactor. Stable atoms of the target element are bombarded with neutrons; the resultant atoms are usually, but not always, isotopic with (that is have the same atomic number as, and are chemically identical to) the target element, and have an excess of neutrons. They tend, therefore, to try to return to a stable configuration by reducing the number of neutrons in the nucleus. A radioactive disintegration takes place, the end result being effectively that a neutron is 'changed into a proton'. The balance of charge is maintained by the emission of an electron, or β-particle. The atomic number is therefore increased by 1, and the new nuclide belongs to an element one place higher in the Periodic Table. For example, tritium is the third isotope of hydrogen; it does not occur naturally but is a radioactive nuclide which is produced by irradiating stable ^2H with neutrons. It decays by β-emission to helium-3 (^3He). The following equations show the processes of production and radioactive decay, and demonstrate the conservation of number of heavy particles, and of electrical charge.

Production: $^{2}_{1}H$	$+ \, ^{1}n$	$\rightarrow \, ^{3}_{1}H$
(hydrogen-2 or deuterium)	(neutron)	(hydrogen-3 or tritium)

Radioactive decay: $^{3}_{1}H \rightarrow \, ^{3}_{2}He$	$+ \, e^{\nearrow}$
(helium)	(β-particle)

The maximum energy of the β-particle is 0.018 MeV

The half-life of the nuclide ^{3}H is 12.26 years

Radioactive phosphorus-32 is produced by the irradiation of stable phosphorus-31 with neutrons, and decays by β-emission to sulphur-32.

Production: $^{31}_{15}P + \, ^{1}n \rightarrow \, ^{32}_{15}P$

Radioactive decay: $^{32}_{15}P \rightarrow \, ^{32}_{16}S + e^{\nearrow}$ (β-particle)

The maximum energy of the β-particles is 1.71 MeV

The half-life of the nuclide ^{32}P is 14.4 days

Positron emission. This is a primary radioactive decay process in which a positron (β^{+}) is emitted. This type of decay usually occurs in radioactive nuclides produced in a cyclotron, one of the machines which produce high-energy protons or deuterons with which to bombard a target element. Stable atoms bombarded with protons or deuterons are transformed into nuclides which are not usually isotopic with the target element, and often have a deficiency of neutrons. They tend, therefore, to try to return to a stable configuration by increasing the number of neutrons. Radioactive decay takes place with the emission of a positron, and effectively a proton is 'changed into a neutron'. The atomic number is therefore decreased by 1, and the new nuclide belongs to an element one place down in the Periodic Table. For example, radioactive oxygen is produced by the irradiation of nitrogen with deuterons. It decays by β^{+}-emission to stable nitrogen.

Production: $^{14}_{7}N + \, ^{2}_{1}H \rightarrow \, ^{15}_{8}O + \, ^{1}n$

Radioactive decay: $^{15}_{8}O \rightarrow \, ^{15}_{7}N + e^{\nearrow}$ (positron)

The maximum energy of the positron is 1.7 MeV

The half-life of the nuclide ^{15}O is 2 minutes

It may be pointed out at this stage that Nature has not been very cooperative with regard to providing useful radioactive isotopes of the biologically important elements carbon, oxygen and nitrogen. The only known radioisotopes of these elements have been impractical because they have half-lives which are either too short (minutes or seconds) or too long (hundreds of years), or emit radiation which cannot be detected outside the body. In recent years applications using very short-lived nuclides have been developed at centres with an on-site cyclotron.

Another example of positron-emission is carbon-11. In naturally occurring carbon there are three isotopes: ^{12}C, ^{13}C, and a trace of ^{14}C which is radioactive. A second radioactive isotope, ^{11}C, does not occur naturally but is cyclotron-produced. These four isotopes of carbon are shown in Table 10.2.

^{14}C can also be produced artificially in a nuclear reactor by bombardment of nitrogen with neutrons. It decays by β-emission.

Production: $^{14}_{7}N + {}^{1}n \rightarrow {}^{14}_{6}C + {}^{1}_{1}H$ (proton)

Radioactive decay: $^{14}_{6}C \rightarrow {}^{14}_{7}N + e^{\nearrow}$ (β-particle)

The maximum energy of the β-particles is 0.159 MeV

The half-life of the nuclide ^{14}C is 5760 years

The fact that ^{14}C occurs naturally in all living material has been used to establish 'carbon-dating' of archaeological specimens. The proportion of ^{14}C in living material is exactly maintained at 10^{-10}%, but when the plant or animal dies, the radioactive decay of ^{14}C causes the ^{14}C content to decrease. By accurate measurement of the proportion of ^{14}C in a specimen it is possible to calculate the age of that specimen; e.g. in 5760 years the ^{14}C content will be reduced to one-half (that is to 0.5×10^{-10}%).

Table 10.2 *Isotopes of carbon*

Nuclide	Nucleus contains: Protons	Nucleus contains: Neutrons	Present in carbon in living organic material	Stable or radioactive
^{11}C	6	5	No; artificially produced	Radioactive
^{12}C	6	6	Yes; 98.89%	Stable
^{13}C	6	7	Yes; 1.11%	Stable
^{14}C	6	8	Yes; 10^{-10}% (also artificially produced)	Radioactive

^{11}C, by contrast, is cyclotron-produced by bombardment of boron with deuterons, and decays by positron-emission.

Production: $^{10}_{5}B + ^{2}_{1}H \rightarrow ^{11}_{6}C + ^{1}n$

Radioactive decay: $^{11}_{6}C \rightarrow ^{11}_{5}B + e^{\nearrow}$ (positron)

The maximum energy of the β-particles is 0.97 MeV

The half life of ^{11}C is 20 minutes

Radioactive decay by positron-emission is always associated with γ-radiation of energy 0.51 MeV. This is because the positron is an unstable particle; almost immediately after emission from the nucleus it is annihilated in combination with an electron, and is transformed into two units (photons) of γ-radiation known as annihilation radiation. In accordance with the law of conservation of mass and energy, the energy of each photon is equivalent to the mass of one electron ($0.00055 m_u = 0.51$ MeV), and the two γ-ray quanta proceed in opposite directions. This phenomenon is utilised in positron scanners and gamma cameras.

Electron capture (or K-capture). This is the fourth primary mode of radioactive decay. It is a process whereby one of the orbital electrons of the atom is captured into the nucleus, thereby effectively changing a proton into a neutron. This mode of decay usually occurs in cyclotron-produced, neutron-deficient radioactive nuclides, but may also occur in nuclides produced by neutron irradiation. As with positron-emission, the resulting nuclide belongs to an element one place down in the Periodic Table. The removal of one of the orbital electrons from the outer atom, usually from the innermost or 'K' shell, leaves the atom in an excited state, i.e. a state of higher energy than normal. The atom reverts to its normal energy state by the emission of characteristic X-radiation. It should be noted that the X-radiation is that associated with the 'daughter element', that is with the atom produced as a result of the radioactive disintegration by electron capture; examples are given below. The decay of a nuclide by electron capture is, therefore, detected by the characteristic radiation of the daughter element. Chromium-51 can be produced in two ways, by neutron or by deuteron bombardment. It decays by electron capture to form vanadium (^{51}V), which then reverts to its normal or ground-state energy with the emission of the characteristic X-radiation of vanadium.

Production:
by neutron bombardment $^{50}_{24}Cr + {}^{1}n \rightarrow {}^{51}_{24}Cr$
by deuteron bombardment $^{51}_{23}V + {}^{2}_{1}H \rightarrow {}^{51}_{24}Cr + 2\,{}^{1}n$

Decay: $^{51}_{24}Cr + e \rightarrow {}^{51}_{23}V$ (excited state)
$\downarrow$
$^{51}_{23}V$ (ground state) + V-characteristic radiation

The energies of the X-rays are 0.0049–0.0054 MeV

The half-life of ^{51}Cr is 27.8 days

Gamma-radiation
The majority of radionuclides decay in such a way that only part of the available energy of the primary processes is carried by the charged particles. The product, or daughter, nucleus is usually formed with an energy higher than that of its ground state, and it reverts to its ground-state energy almost instantaneously, with the emission of γ-radiation of appropriate energy.

For example cobalt-60 disintegrates by β-emission to form nickel-60, with associated γ-ray emission. The disintegration scheme, or decay scheme as it is often called, is represented in Fig. 10.1. The horizontal levels indicate the energy level of the product nucleus above its ground state, and the vertical lines the γ-radiation emitted as the nucleus reduces its energy.

Primary mode of disintegration: β-decay

Maximum energy: β_1 0.31 MeV (99.8%)
β_2 1.48 MeV (0.02%)

Gamma radiation: γ_1 1.17 MeV
γ_2 1.33 MeV

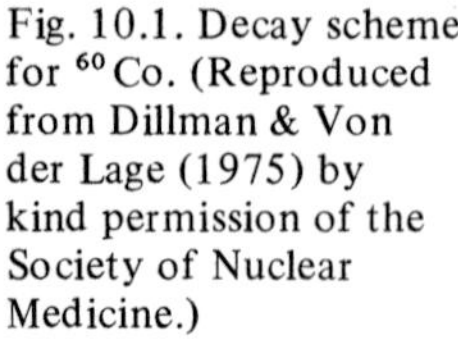
Fig. 10.1. Decay scheme for ^{60}Co. (Reproduced from Dillman & Von der Lage (1975) by kind permission of the Society of Nuclear Medicine.)

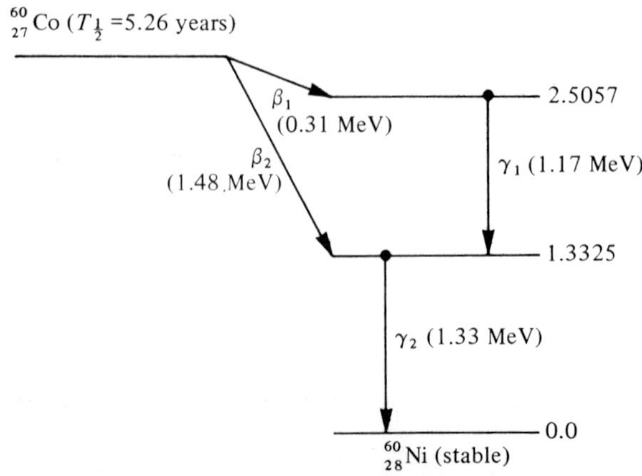

Metastable states and isomeric transitions

Occasionally the product nucleus from one of the above primary processes is in a metastable state, i.e. decays to its ground-state energy by emitting γ-radiation, with a detectable half-life which is often a fraction of a second but may be as long as several hours. The metastable state of a nuclide is denoted by the letter 'm' after the mass number, and the process of its decay is referred to as isomeric decay. An important example of this is technetium-99m (^{99m}Tc), which is formed by the β-decay of molybdenum-99 and decays according to the scheme shown in Fig. 10.2. Technetium-99m was considered in more detail in Chapter 5.

Complex disintegration schemes

The disintegration schemes of the nuclides considered above are simple, having only one primary mode of decay which takes place in all disintegrations. Many nuclides have very complex schemes, in which β-emission, β^+-emission and electron capture all take place in constant, pre-determined proportions, and γ-rays may follow all three types of transition. An example of such a complex scheme is iodine-126, which decays to both tellurium-126 and xenon-126. Its decay scheme is given in Fig. 10.3.

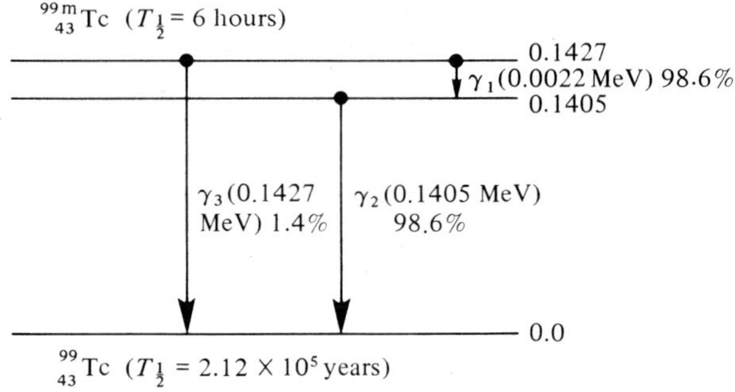

Fig. 10.2. Decay scheme for ^{99m}Tc. (Reproduced from Dillman & Von der Lage (1975) by kind permission of the Society of Nuclear Medicine.)

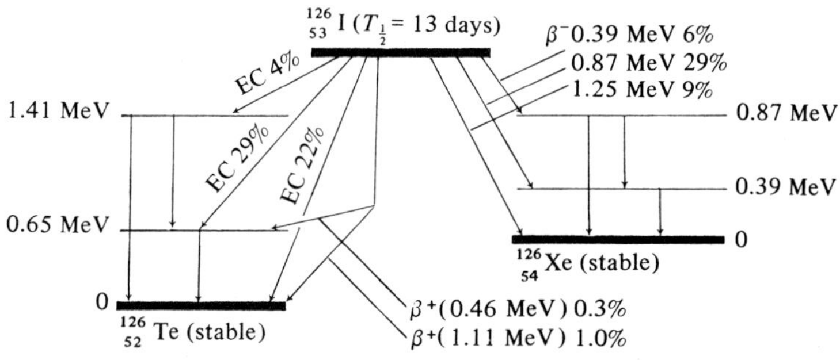

Fig. 10.3. Decay scheme for ^{126}I. (Reproduced from Wilson (1966) by kind permission of The Radiochemical Centre.)

Internal conversion and Auger electrons
It is important to realise that the nuclear disintegration schemes as already outlined do not give the complete picture of radiation emitted. A disintegration scheme gives the primary mode of decay and the associated γ-radiation emitted from the nucleus, but does not include the characteristic radiation of the daughter element when decay is by electron capture. The nuclear decay data is referred to as the input data (Dillman, 1969). As a result of interaction within the electron structure of the atom there may be, in addition, internal conversion electrons, characteristic radiation, and Auger electrons. Internal conversion is the phenomenon whereby the energy of some of the γ-ray photons may be imparted to inner orbital electrons, which are thereby ejected from the atom. There is always characteristic X-radiation associated with electron capture, and there may also be characteristic radiation associated with internal conversion. In some instances the excess energy which produces characteristic X-radiation is transferred to one of the outer electrons, which is thereby ejected; these electrons are referred to as Auger electrons. The complete end-product of emitted radiation is referred to as the output data. From a practical point of view it is important to appreciate that there is, almost invariably, some electron emission associated with every radioactive nuclide, even when the decay scheme shows only γ- or X-radiation, as, for example with ^{99m}Tc. Table 10.3 shows the input data for ^{99m}Tc which correspond to the decay scheme in Fig. 10.2, and also the output data, which are much more complex. Apart from the main Gamma-2 component, of energy 0.1405 MeV, which is present in 88.3% of disintegrations, they include internal conversion electrons and Auger electrons, as well as characteristic X-radiation.

Rate of disintegration

Each radioactive nuclide is characterised by its own disintegration constant. There is no known way of altering this constant. Radioactivity is a purely random process, that is the rate of disintegration is proportional to the number of atoms present. This may be expressed mathematically by the equation

$$A = \frac{\mathrm{d}N}{\mathrm{d}t} = -\lambda N \qquad (10.1)$$

where A = activity, i.e. the rate of disintegration
N = number of atoms present

t = time
λ = disintegration constant
Integrating equation 10.1 gives

$$N = N_0 e^{-\lambda t} \quad (10.2)$$

where N_0 is the number of atoms or molecules present initially.

Table 10.3 *Input and output data for* ^{99m}Tc

Input data[a]

Radiation	% per disintegration	Transition energy (MeV)	Other nuclear parameters
Gamma-1	98.6	0.0022	E3, α very large
Gamma-2	98.6	0.1405	M1, $\alpha_K = 0.10$, K/L = 8.1
Gamma-3	1.4	0.1427	M4, α_K = 29(T), α_L = 9.19(T)

Output data

Radiation (i)	Mean number per disintegration, n_i	Mean energy, $\bar{E}_i$ (MeV)	Δ_i (g-rad μCi^{-1} h^{-1})
Gamma-1	0.00	0.0021	0.0000
M int. con. electron, gamma-1	0.986	0.0017	0.0036
Gamma-2	0.883	0.1405	0.2643
K int. con. electron, gamma-2	0.0883	0.1195	0.0225
L int. con. electron, gamma-2	0.0109	0.1377	0.0032
M int. con. electron, gamma-2	0.0036	0.1401	0.0011
Gamma-3	0.0003	0.1427	0.0001
K int. con. electron, gamma-3	0.0096	0.1217	0.0025
L int. con. electron, gamma-3	0.0030	0.1399	0.0009
M int. con. electron, gamma-3	0.0010	0.1423	0.0003
K α-1 X-rays	0.0431	0.0184	0.0017
K α-2 X-rays	0.0216	0.0183	0.0008
K β-1 X-rays	0.0103	0.0206	0.0005
K β-2 X-rays	0.0018	0.0210	0.0001
L X-rays	0.0081	0.0024	0.0000
KLL Auger electron	0.0149	0.0155	0.0005
KLX Auger electron	0.0055	0.0178	0.0002
KXY Auger electron	0.0007	0.0202	0.0000
LMM Auger electron	0.106	0.0019	0.0004
MXY Auger electron	1.23	0.0004	0.0010

From Dillman & Von der Lage (1975).
[a]From Lederer *et al.* (1967). (T), theoretical value.

Since

$$A = -\lambda N$$

$$A = A_0 e^{-\lambda t} \tag{10.3}$$

where A_0 is the initial activity.

Equation 10.2 states mathematically that the number of atoms present at any time t is an exponential function determined by the disintegration constant (or decay constant), λ, of the nuclide. It may be written alternatively as

$$\log_e \frac{N}{N_0} = -\lambda t \tag{10.4}$$

λ is expressed in reciprocal time, that is seconds^{-1}, minutes^{-1}, hours^{-1}, days^{-1}, or years^{-1} as appropriate, and the time t must be expressed in the same unit. It is usual to specify the disintegration rate of a nuclide by its half-life ($T_{\frac{1}{2}}$) rather than by its decay constant. The half-life is defined as the time in which the activity, or number of radioactive atoms, of the nuclide falls to one-half of its original value.

From equation 10.4 and putting t equal to $T_{\frac{1}{2}}$,

$$\log_e (\tfrac{1}{2}) = -\lambda T_{\frac{1}{2}}$$

$$\text{i.e. } T_{\frac{1}{2}} = \frac{0.693}{\lambda} \quad \text{or,} \quad \lambda = \frac{0.693}{T_{\frac{1}{2}}} \quad \text{since } \log_e 2 = 0.693$$

Substituting in equation 10.3

$$\log_e \frac{A}{A_0} = \frac{-0.693\, t}{T_{\frac{1}{2}}} \tag{10.5}$$

Since logarithms to the base 10 are more commonly used, the following equation is more practical:

$$\log_{10} \frac{A}{A_0} = \frac{-[\log_{10} 2]\, t}{T_{\frac{1}{2}}} = \frac{-0.3010t}{T_{\frac{1}{2}}} \tag{10.6}$$

If the decay of activity of any single radioactive nuclide is plotted against time, on a linear scale, according to equation 10.3, an exponential curve will result, theoretically reaching zero at infinite time. Decay curves plotted in this way for five of the iodine isotopes are shown in Fig. 10.4(*a*). It is more instructive to plot the logarithm of activity against time; according to equation 10.6 the result is a straight line of slope $0.3010/T_{\frac{1}{2}}$ (Fig. 10.4*b*).

Units of activity

The old unit of activity is the curie (Ci), which is defined as the amount of a radioactive substance which gives rise to 3.7×10^{10} disintegrations per second. The curie was chosen for the unit of radioactivity in connection with radium, in honour of the Curies, who discovered the element. It was intended to be the activity of 1 gram of radium, in equilibrium with all its decay products. The curie is a large unit, and it is the millicurie (mCi), the amount of radioactivity which gives rise to 3.7×10^7 disintegrations per second, and the microcurie (μCi), which gives rise

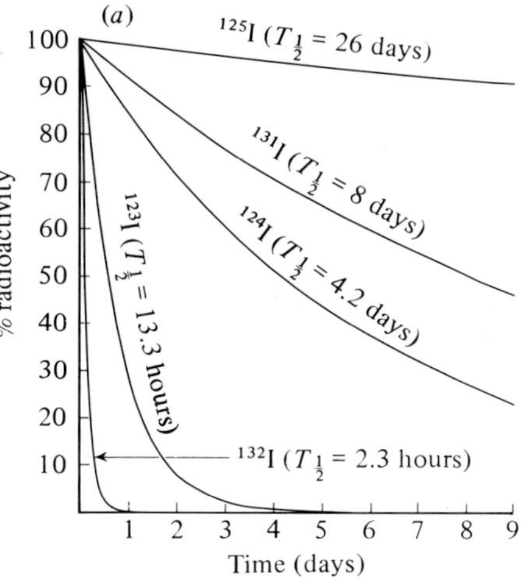

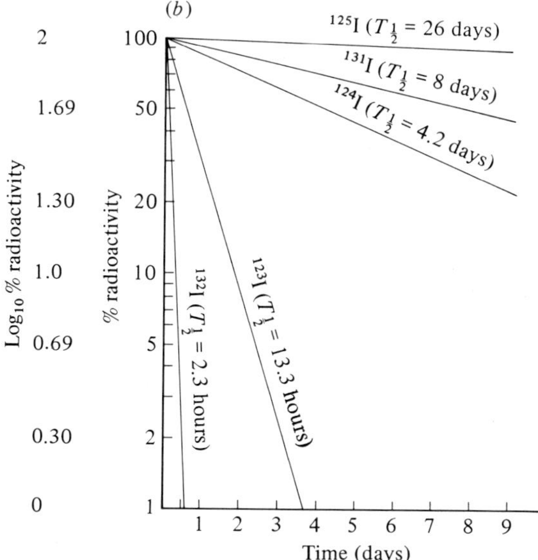

Fig. 10.4. Exponential decay of four isotopes of iodine, plotted on (*a*) linear and (*b*) log-linear scales.

to 3.7×10^4 disintegrations per second, that are commonly used in medical work. The new SI unit of activity which was adopted in June 1975 is the becquerel (Bq). (The name becquerel is in honour of Henri Becquerel who discovered radioactivity in 1896.) It is the rate of spontaneous nuclear transformation, and is expressed in reciprocal seconds (seconds^{-1}): that is, 1 becquerel corresponds to 1 disintegration per second. It is therefore a very much smaller unit than even the microcurie. Conversion factors are given in Table 10.4.

The old units of curies, millicuries and microcuries are to be gradually abandoned over a period of not less than 10 years,* and to be replaced by the becquerel. Although common usage has made that rather strange unit the curie acceptable, the new unit, being simply 1 disintegration per second, is a fundamental unit, and students of the future will not have to memorise the curious figure of 3.7×10^{10} disintegrations per second. However, with the current levels of administered dose it will mean working in kilobecquerels (kBq), megabecquerels (MBq) even gigabecquerels (GBq), as shown in Table 10.4. In this book both the old unit, the curie, and its SI equivalent are used throughout.

Specific activity

The specific activity of a sample of radioactivity is the activity per unit mass of an element, or compound, containing one of its radioactive isotopes. The maximum possible specific activity is that of a pure (or 'carrier-free') nuclide when all the atoms or

Table 10.4 *Curies and becquerels: conversions*

(a) Conversion of curies to becquerels		
1 μCi	3.7×10^4 Bq	37 kBq
10 μCi	3.7×10^5 Bq	370 kBq
100 μCi	3.7×10^6 Bq	3.7 MBq
1 mCi	3.7×10^7 Bq	37 MBq
10 mCi	3.7×10^8 Bq	370 MBq
100 mCi	3.7×10^9 Bq	3.7 GBq
1 Ci	3.7×10^{10} Bq	37 GBq
(b) Conversion of becquerels to curies		
1 Bq	2.7×10^{-11} Ci	27 pCi
1 kBq	2.7×10^{-8} Ci	27 nCi
1 MBq	2.7×10^{-5} Ci	27 μCi
1 GBq	2.7×10^{-2} Ci	27 mCi

*See 'Note added in proof' on p. 186.

molecules present are those of the radionuclide in question.

One gram of an element contains $(6.02 \times 10^{23})/W$ atoms, where 6.02×10^{23} is Avogadro's number and W is the atomic weight of the element. From equation 10.1 and the definition of the curie, it follows that the number of curies in 1 g of a pure radionuclide, i.e. the maximum specific activity, is

$$\frac{\lambda(6.02 \times 10^{23})}{W(3.7 \times 10^{10})} \text{ Ci g}^{-1}$$

$$= \frac{0.693}{T_{\frac{1}{2}}W} \frac{6.02 \times 10^{23}}{3.7 \times 10^{10}} \text{ Ci g}^{-1} \text{ if } T_{\frac{1}{2}} \text{ is in seconds}$$

$$= \frac{1.128 \times 10^{13}}{T_{\frac{1}{2}}W} \text{ Ci g}^{-1} \qquad (10.7)$$

The number of becquerels in 1 g of a pure radionuclide is

$$\frac{4.17 \times 10^{23}}{T_{\frac{1}{2}}W} \text{ Bq g}^{-1} \qquad (10.8)$$

From equations 10.7 and 10.8 it is possible to calculate the amount of, for example, ^{99m}Tc in 10 mCi (370 MBq) of carrier-free material:

$$W = 99$$

$$T_{\frac{1}{2}} = 6 \text{ hours} = 2.16 \times 10^4 \text{ seconds}$$

Therefore amount of ^{99m}Tc in 10 mCi (370 MBq)

$$= \frac{(2.16 \times 10^4)}{(1.128 \times 10^{13})} \frac{99}{100} \text{g} = 2 \text{ ng}$$

If a radionuclide contains stable atoms or molecules of the element or compound in question, it is said to contain carrier.

Summary

The properties which fully characterise a radioactive nuclide are:

(1) Chemical symbol and atomic number, that is, number of protons.

(2) Atomic mass number, that is, number of protons and neutrons.

(3) Mode of disintegration, types of radiation and their energy.

(4) Decay constant or half-life.

To specify a particular sample of radioactive material the following information is necessary:

(1) Chemical symbol and mass number.
(2) The activity in millicuries or microcuries (in SI units, becquerels).
(3) The volume, and activity per unit volume.
(4) The reference date and, with short-lived nuclides, the reference time at which the radioactive content applies.
(5) The specific activity.

Any radioactive material being dispensed must immediately be given a label bearing the radioactive symbol and the first four items above.

References

Dillman, L.T. & Von der Lage, F.C. (1975). *Radionuclide Decay Schemes and Nuclear Parameters for Use in Radiation-dose Estimations.* nm/mird pamphlet No. 10. New York: Society of Nuclear Medicine.

Lederer, M., Hollander, J.M., & Perlman, I. (1967). *Table of Isotopes*, 6th ed. New York: Wiley.

Wilson, B.J. (ed.) (1966). *The Radiochemical Manual*, 2nd ed. Amersham: The Radiochemical Centre.

Note added in proof

The EC draft directive (p. 208) recommends that 1985 be the date on which the old units of radioactivity, the roentgen, rad, rem and curie, cease to be authorised for use for official purposes throughout the EEC.

11. Radiation exposure, absorbed dose, and protection

Nature of radiation and properties of ionising radiations

The term ionising radiation is a general one applied to radiations which are detected by virtue of the ionisations they produce in their passage through matter. It includes gamma (γ)-radiation, X-radiation, and particulate radiation such as β-radiation, neutrons, and beams of protons or deuterons. Charged particulate radiations produce ionisation directly; γ- and X-radiation produce ionisation only via secondary-electron production, and neutrons via protons.

β-radiation

β-radiation, as described in Chapter 10, is a stream of electrons, and one can visualise these tiny particles moving through, for example, air or water, and colliding with the atoms. During one of these collisions an outer electron may be knocked off an atom, leaving a positively charged atom, or positive ion; this together with the free electron or a negative ion forms an ion pair. The β-particle will continue along its path producing ionisation until it has expended all its energy, and comes to the end of its path. By this process the energy of the β-radiation is absorbed by the medium through which it passes, and it is this energy deposited in the material that is responsible for radiation damage. Radiation dose is measured in terms of energy absorption per unit mass of tissue.

The density of ion pairs produced, and therefore the radiation damage, is dependent on several factors. Primarily it depends on the velocity and charge of the particle; a proton will be more densely ionising than a β-particle of the same energy, and an α-particle (helium nucleus) of that energy will be even more densely ionising. Fig. 11.1 shows diagrammatic representations of the ionising tracks of an α-particle, a β-particle, and the secondary electrons produced by the passage of a γ-ray. It is evident that the greater the ion density the sooner the ionising particle will expend all its energy and the shorter will be its length of path, or range. The range of an α-particle is very short compared with that of a β-particle of equal energy. The range of any specific type of particulate radiation is dependent on its energy.

This energy is commonly expressed in million-electron-volts (MeV) or kilo-electron-volts (keV). The values for the ranges of β-particles in air, water and tissue may be found in the National Bureau of Standards Circular 577 and Supplement (NBS, 1956/8). Some ranges in air, water and tissue for β-ray energies commonly encountered in medical work are given in Table 11.1. It will be

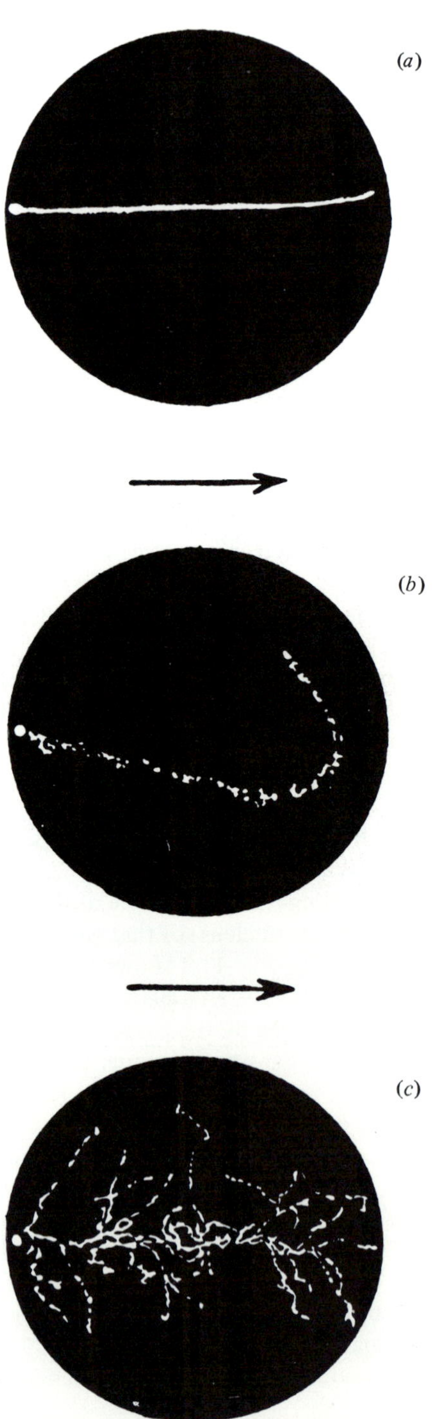

Fig. 11.1. Diagrammatic representation of ionising tracks of (*a*) an α-particle, (*b*) a β-particle, and (*c*) the secondary electrons produced by an γ-ray.

noted that although the ranges in air are appreciable the ranges in tissue are very short. The energies and ranges given are the maximum values. The β-radiation given off by any radioactive nuclide covers a complete range of energies from zero up to the maximum energy, which is specific for that nuclide. The average energy of the radiation is approximately one-third of the maximum value.

X-radiation and γ-radiation
X- and γ-radiation have already been referred to in Chapter 10 as being emitted during radioactive disintegration of an atom. They are electromagnetic radiations of the same nature as visible light and radio waves, differing only in their quantum energy, or wavelength. The distinction between γ- and X-radiation relates to their origin. The term γ-radiation is reserved for nuclear radiation which is given off when the nucleus of an atom is in an excited energy state and returns to its ground state with the emission of radiation. Characteristic X-radiation is the term used for atomic radiation which is given off when an atom, which is in an excited energy state due to a vacancy in one of its electron orbits, returns to its ground state by rearrangement of the orbital electrons to fill the vacancy. γ-radiation is usually of higher energy than characteristic X-radiation, being more comparable with the radiation used in radiotherapy, whereas the characteristic X-radiation is more comparable with that used in diagnostic radiography. From the point of view of interaction with matter and radiation exposure they may be considered together, and will be referred to collectively as γ-radiation, except where the text refers specifically to X-radiation.

Table 11.1 *Maximum ranges of β-particles*

		Range				
Nuclide	Energy (MeV)	Air (cm)	Glass (mm)	Polystyrene (mm)	Lead (mm)	Water or tissue (mm)
^{3}H	0.018	0.7	–	0.007	–	0.007
^{99m}Tc	0.12 (internal conversion)	20	–	0.2	–	0.2
^{14}C	0.155	28	–	0.14	–	0.29
^{131}I	0.33	≈ 100	–	1.1	–	1.0
	0.61	≈ 200	–	2.0	–	2.0
^{198}Au	1.0	≈ 400	1.6	4.5	1	4.4
^{32}P	1.71	≈ 500	2.8	8.0	1	8.2

γ-radiation is different from particulate radiation in that it cannot be detected directly, but only by virtue of the secondary electrons it produces when it traverses and interacts with matter such as air, water or tissue. This phenomenon was first demonstrated in the elegant cloud-chamber experiments of C.T.R. Wilson. It was known that when a chamber of saturated water vapour is made to expand suddenly, a cooling effect occurs which causes the water vapour to condense and form droplets on any particles, e.g. dust, which are present. Wilson directed a beam of X-radiation through such a cloud-chamber and his photographs showed the electron tracks produced. One of his original photographs is reproduced in Fig. 11.2; the direction of the X-ray beam is from left to right, and the tortuous tracks of individual secondary electrons can be seen, radiating in all directions from the direction of the beam. Thus the energy of the X-ray beam is absorbed into the medium which it traverses, via the production of secondary electrons and subsequently of ion pairs.

Inverse square law. Like all electromagnetic radiation, the intensity of γ-radiation from a point source is subject to the inverse square law. The emission of γ-radiation is isotropic, that is equal in all directions. It follows that the area over which the radiation energy is distributed increases as the square of the distance from a point source, and consequently the intensity of radiation, expressed as energy per unit area, varies inversely as the square of the distance. This is shown diagrammatically in Fig. 11.3, and may be expressed mathematically as

Fig. 11.2. Photograph of a cloud-chamber experiment showing electron tracks. (Reproduced from S.G. Starling (1941), *Electricity and Magnetism for Degree Students*, 2nd edn, by kind permission of the publishers Longman Ltd.)

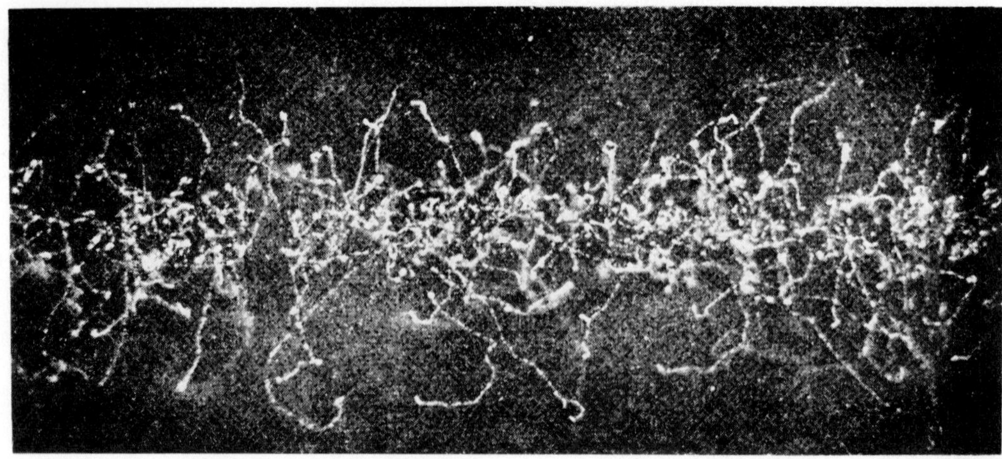

$$I \propto \frac{1}{r^2} \tag{11.1}$$

where I = exposure rate due to a point source
r = the distance from that source

Attenuation coefficient. As γ-radiation traverses any medium, its interaction with the material of the medium, such as air, water or tissue, causes reduction in its intensity. This effect is referred to as attenuation. The attenuation of γ-radiation from any specified nuclide in any specified medium is dependent only on the intensity of radiation and therefore is an exponential process, which may be expressed mathematically as

$$\frac{\mathrm{d}I}{\mathrm{d}x} \propto I \text{ or } \frac{\mathrm{d}I}{\mathrm{d}x} = \mu I \tag{11.2}$$

where x = thickness of the medium traversed
μ = total linear attenuation coefficient and is a property of the medium and the energy of the γ-radiation

Integrating equation 11.2,

$$I = \mathrm{e}^{-\mu x} \text{ const}$$

but when $x = 0, I = I_0$, and therefore

$$I = I_0 \mathrm{e}^{-\mu x} \tag{11.3}$$

Values of μ for many different materials, for energies from 0.01 MeV to 10 MeV may be found in the National Bureau of Standards Circular 583 (NBS, 1957).

More commonly, attenuation is expressed in terms of a half-value-layer, $x_{\frac{1}{2}}$, that is the thickness of the specified material which is required to reduce the intensity to one-half its initial value. From equation 11.3 and the above definition:

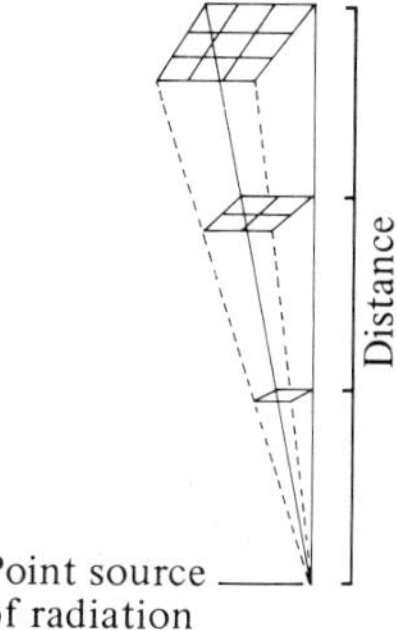

Fig. 11.3. Illustration of the inverse square law.

$$x_{\frac{1}{2}} = \frac{\log_e 2}{\mu} \tag{11.4}$$

Some typical values for the attenuation of γ-radiation commonly encountered in medical work, in air, water, tissue and lead are given in Table 11.2.

Below energies of 1.02 MeV there are two components of the attenuation coefficient, one being due to Compton scattering and absorption and the other to photoelectric absorption. In Compton scattering only part of the energy of the incident photon is imparted to the secondary electron and truly absorbed. During this process the photon loses energy and suffers a change in direction, thus producing scattered or degraded γ-radiation, and secondary electrons which are of lesser energy than the incident radiation and are known as Compton electrons. Scattered radiation has an important bearing on problems of collimation, as was discussed in Chapter 7. By contrast, in photoelectric absorption all the energy of the incident γ-ray photon is imparted to the secondary electron, which is known as a photoelectron. The relative value of the two coefficients is highly dependent on the atomic number of the absorbing medium, as well as on the energy of the incident radiation, since the photoelectric absorption coefficient is proportional to Z^4 while that for Compton scattering varies little with Z. This is why lead, which has an atomic number of 82, has such a high attenuation coefficient at low energies.

Table 11.2 *Half-value layers (HVL) for γ-radiation*

Energy (MeV)	Nuclide with principal γ-ray of this order	HVL in water or tissue (cm)	HVL in lead (mm)
0.01	–	0.13	–
0.027	^{125}I	1.39	0.02
0.1	–	4.0	0.1
0.14	^{99m}Tc	4.5	0.25
0.3	^{131}I (0.36 MeV and 0.64 MeV)	5.8	1.6
0.55	^{18}F (annihilation radiation)	7.5	0.5
0.75	^{99}Mo (0.74 MeV and 0.78 MeV)	8.3	0.7
1.0	^{24}Na (1.37 MeV and 2.75 MeV)	10	1
2.0		12	1.3

Radiation exposure, energy absorption and absorbed radiation dose

Hazards of exposure to ionising radiations

Any exposure to radiation is assumed to entail a risk of deleterious effects. These risks have been considered by the International Commission on Radiological Protection, who recommended maximum permissible doses (MPD) (ICRP, 1965), for members of the public and for radiation workers. The 1965 recommendations were amended in 1969 and in 1971. These amended ICRP values were adopted in the European Communities (EC) Council Directive (1976). More recently the ICRP has reviewed its basic recommendations in the light of new information which has emerged during the last decade, and has published new recommendations (ICRP, 1977*b*). The ICRP now recommends a system of dose limitation, and ICRP Publication 26 (ICRP, 1977*b*) gives dose equivalent limits (DEL) for radiation workers and members of the public. The DEL supersede the MPD in ICRP Publication 9 (ICRP, 1965), but not necessarily the recommendations of other bodies, even those with which the ICRP maintains close working contacts.

Both sets of recommendations are given in Table 11.3. They apply to radiation arising from sources outside the body or from radioactive material within the body, and are concerned entirely with exposures other than those received by patients in the course of medical procedures. The values in ICRP Publication 9 were given in rems, but have been converted to sieverts in Table 11.3 for purposes of comparison. Corresponding values in rems, as originally published, are also given. Definitions of rem and sievert are given on p. 197.

It will be noticed that there is a distinction between stochastic and non-stochastic effects. Stochastic effects are those for which the probability of an effect occurring, rather than its severity, is regarded as a function of dose, without threshold. At the dose range involved in radiation protection, hereditary effects are considered to be stochastic, as is also carcinogenesis. Non-stochastic effects are those for which the severity of the effect varies with the dose, and for which a threshold may therefore occur; some are specific to particular tissues, as in the case of cataract of the lens, non-malignant damage to the skin, and cell depletion in the bone marrow. The lowest DEL, whether stochastic or non-stochastic, is the limiting value.

Comparison of the two sets of values shows that the DEL for the whole body is the same as the old MPD. While the old MPD

Table 11.3 *Dose equivalent limits (DEL) in mSv in a year given or implied by ICRP Publication 26 with comparative limits (MPD) in ICRP Publication 9*

	Worker				Member of the public[a]			
			MPD				MPD	
Tissue/organ	Stochastic[b]	Non-stochastic[b]	mSv	rem	Stochastic[b]	Non-stochastic[b]	mSv	rem
Whole body	50[c]	–	50	5	5[d]	–	5	0.5
Tissues/organs irradiated singly:								
Gonads	200	(500)	50	5	20	(50)	5	0.5
Breast	330	(500)	150	15	33	(50)	15	1.5
Red bone marrow	417	(500)	50	5	42	(50)	5	0.5
Lung	417	(500)	150	15	42	(50)	15	1.5
Thyroid	(1670)	500	300	30	(167)	50	30	3.0
Bone surfaces	(1670)	500	–		(167)	50	–	
Lens	–	300	150	15	–	50	15	1.5
Other single organ	(833)	500	150	15	(83)	50	15	1.5
Bone	–	–	300	30	–		30	3.0
Skin	–	500	300	30	–	50	30	3.0
Hands and forearms	–	–	750	75	–	–	75	7.5
Feet and ankles	–	–	750	75	–	–	75	7.5
Planned special exposure								
Single	2 × DEL		2 × DEL					
Lifetime	5 × DEL		5 × DEL					
Pregnant women: after diagnosis of pregnancy	0.3 × DEL *pro rata*[e]		10[f]					

From NRPB-R63 (1977). *Recommendations of the ICRP. ICRP Publication 26: A Summary*. Harwell: NRPB.

[a]No DEL for populations is recommended but application of the DELs for individuals, as well as observance of the Commission's general principles, is likely to ensure that the average dose-equivalent to a population will not exceed 0.5 mSv per year. (The genetic dose limit in *ICRP Publication 9* was 50 mSv in 30 years.)

[b]The DEL is the stochastic or the non-stochastic limit, whichever is the lower. (The higher value is shown in brackets.)

[c]This limit applies both to uniform irradiation of the whole body and to the weighted mean of the doses to individual tissues. For external irradiation, when the dose distribution is unknown, the limit applies to the deep dose equivalent index.

[d]As exposures at the DEL are not likely to be repeated over many years, this limit is likely to ensure that the lifetime dose to a member of the public will not exceed 1 mSv per year.

[e]For example, 0.175 × DEL in 7 months.

[f][illegible]

for hands and forearms (750 mSv) was greater than that for the skin generally (300 mSv), there is no specified DEL for hands and forearms and that for the skin (500 mSv) applies; thus the limit for hand exposure is reduced from 750 mSv to 500 mSv.

The ICRP has also considered separately the radiation doses caused by radioactive material deposited in the body, and made recommendations for maximum permissible body burden (MPBB) and maximum permissible concentrations in air (MPCa) and in drinking water (MPCw) for different radionuclides (ICRP, 1959, 1964). The EEC Council Directive has laid down values of intake and concentration of radionuclides in air, to be used in implementing the requirements for MPD. The ICRP now uses a system of annual limits of intake (ALI); these are calculated by their Committee 2 to be such that the recommended DEL are not exceeded (ICRP, 1977*a*). A further report on the limits for intakes of radionuclides by workers is in preparation (ICRP, 1979).

The radiation dose to patients receiving radioactive nuclides for diagnostic purposes is another matter and needs to be weighed against the benefit of the investigation to the patient. In order to do this, the radiation dose is calculated as accurately as possible, with the information available, for each type of investigation (ICRP, 1971).

To get a sense of proportion with regard to radiation hazards it is necessary to know something about the radiation exposure and radiation dose involved. Radiation exposure relates to quantity of β- or γ-radiation, and is measured by the degree of ionisation produced in air. Radiation dose is measured in terms of energy absorption, and may result from radiation arising outside the body (external radiation), in which case it is directly proportional to radiation exposure, from radiation arising inside the body (internal radiation) due to radionuclides deposited in the body, or from contamination due to radionuclides deposited on the skin.

Units

The old unit of radiation exposure is the roentgen (R). The roentgen was first defined in 1940 as a unit of X- or γ-radiation such that the associated corpuscular emission per 0.00129 g of air (1 cm^3 at NTP) produces, in air, ions carrying one electrostatic unit (e.s.u.) of quantity of electricity of either sign; it is exactly defined in terms of the SI unit for exposure as 2.58×10^{-4} coulombs per kilogram ($C\ kg^{-1}$) ($1\ C = 3 \times 10^9$ e.s.u.). The new

SI unit of exposure will be C kg^{-1} but has not yet been named. The definition of the roentgen requires that it is measured in air.

The old unit of absorbed radiation dose is the rad, which was defined as being equivalent to the absorption of 100 ergs (or 10^{-5} joules) per gram of tissue. The new SI unit is the gray (Gy), which is defined as the energy absorption of 1 joule per kilogram (J kg^{-1}). The rad is equal to 10^{-2} Gy.

The relationship between exposure (X) and absorbed dose (D_m) in a medium is given by

$$D_m \approx X\, w\, n\, (\mu/\rho)_m \,/\, (\mu/\rho)_a \qquad (11.5)$$

where w = mean energy expended in air per ion pair formed,
$\approx 33.7\,(1.602 \times 10^{-19})$ J, over a wide range of energies,
$\approx 54.00 \times 10^{-19}$ J
n = number of ion pairs produced per unit mass for unit exposure
$(\mu/\rho)_m$ and $(\mu/\rho)_a$ = mass energy absorption coefficients for the material and air, respectively, for the mean energy of radiation

In old units, D_m is in rads, X is in roentgens, and n is the number of ion pairs produced per gram per roentgen, which, by definition, since the electronic charge is 4.8×10^{-10} e.s.u., equals

$$\frac{1/(4.8 \times 10^{-10})}{0.001293}$$

Therefore,

$$D_m \approx \frac{X(54.00 \times 10^{-19})\,(\mu/\rho)_m}{(4.8 \times 10^{-10})0.001293\,(\mu/\rho)_a}\ \text{J g}^{-1}$$

$$\approx X(0.87 \times 10^{-5})\,(\mu/\rho)_m \,/\, (\mu/\rho)_a \ \text{J g}^{-1}$$

$$\approx X\, 0.87\, (\mu/\rho)_m \,/\, (\mu/\rho)_a \ \text{rad} \qquad (11.6)$$

In SI units, D_m is in grays, X is in coulombs per kilogram, and n is the number of ion pairs produced per coulomb per kilogram, which, since the electronic charge is 1.602×10^{-19} C, equals $1/(1.602 \times 10^{-19})$. Therefore,

$$D_m \approx X\, 33.7\, (\mu/\rho)_m \,/\, (\mu/\rho)_a \ \text{Gy} \qquad (11.7)$$

The ratio $(\mu/\rho)_m \,/\, (\mu/\rho)_a$ is almost constant at a value of 1.1 for muscle, at energies between 200 and 2000 keV. It follows from equations 11.6 and 11.7 that the factor relating roentgens to rads, for muscle, at these energies is 0.87×1.1, i.e. 0.96, and that relating coulombs per kilogram to grays is 33.7 × 1.1, i.e. 37.0. Table 11.4 gives the factors relating absorbed dose to exposure (expressed in Gy per C kg^{-1} and in rad per R) for water, bone and muscle for γ-radiation of varying energies. It will be noted that whereas in the old units the absorbed dose in water and muscle is numerically approximately equal to the exposure, over a range of energies, this is not so in SI units.

As shown earlier in this chapter the specific ionisation, and the radiation damage for a given dose, vary with the type of radiation. In order to allow for this, the physical quantity dose-equivalent, measured in rems, was introduced, and a factor used to convert rads to rems. The factor is 1 for X- and γ-radiation. The ICRP have decided to retain the quantity dose-equivalent, to define the new unit as J kg^{-1} and to call it the sievert (Sv), which is equal to 100 rem. It will be numerically equal to the gray for X- and γ-radiation. The dose-equivalent, H, at a point in tissue is given by

$$H = DQN \tag{11.8}$$

where H is in sieverts, D, the absorbed dose, is in grays, Q is the quality factor, and N is the product of all other modifying factors specified by the ICRP. For the time being it is assumed that N equals 1.

The rad, the roentgen and the rem are to be gradually abandoned, together with the curie, but the date when they will cease to be accepted units has not yet been decided.* In this book, therefore, both the old units and their SI equivalents are used.

*See 'Note added in proof' on p. 186.

γ-radiation exposure and absorbed dose from an external source

In considering absorbed dose of γ-radiation from the point of view of radiation protection, it is usually assumed to be from a

Table 11.4 *Factor relating absorbed dose to exposure for photons from 10 keV to 2 MeV under conditions of charged-particle equilibrium*

Photon energy (keV)	Water		Bone		Muscle	
	Gy per C kg^{-1}	rad per R	Gy per C kg^{-1}	rad per R	Gy per C kg^{-1}	rad per R
10	35.0	0.904	140	3.70	34.0	0.877
50	34.7	0.894	134	3.46	34.3	0.885
100	36.9	0.951	56.1	1.45	36.5	0.940
200	37.4	0.965	37.9	0.977	37.0	0.954
2000	37.5	0.966	35.6	0.924	37.0	0.955

From ICRU Recommendations on Dosimetry and Quantitative Concentration in Radiobiology (draft of 22 July 1977, now in press).

source external to the body. The exposure arising from a source may be calculated in roentgens or coulombs per kilogram; the absorbed dose in rads or grays and the dose-equivalent in rems or sieverts may then be calculated.

Each radionuclide has its own disintegration scheme, and each γ-emitting nuclide will give rise to a certain γ-ray exposure which is known as the exposure rate constant (Γ) and is defined as: 'the radiation exposure rate due to a point source of one millicurie of a particular nuclide, at one centimetre, expressed in roentgens per hour'. It can be measured experimentally, or calculated as follows.

For a source of 1 mCi of a nuclide with a 100% emission of γ-rays of mean energy $\bar{E}$ MeV the total energy emitted per second is given as

$$\begin{aligned}\text{Total energy} &= (3.7 \times 10^{7})\bar{E} \text{ MeV per second} \\ &= (3.7 \times 10^{7})\bar{E}(1.602 \times 10^{-13}) \text{ J per second}\end{aligned}$$

Since the emission is isotropic, the energy is uniform over the surface of a sphere of radius 1 cm, i.e. an area of 4π cm^2. Therefore the energy flux at 1 cm from the source per hour

$$= \frac{(3.7 \times 10^{7})\bar{E}(1.602 \times 10^{-13})(3.6 \times 10^{3})}{4\pi}$$

$$= (1.70 \times 10^{-3})\bar{E} \text{ J h}^{-1} \text{ cm}^{-2}$$

The total absorption coefficient for γ-ray photon energies between 0.08 MeV and 2 MeV is approximately constant with a mean value of 0.026 cm^2 g^{-1} air. Therefore the energy absorption rate per gram of air per millicurie

$$= (1.70 \times 10^{-3})\,\bar{E}\,0.026$$

$$= (4.42 \times 10^{-5})\,\bar{E} \text{ J h}^{-1} \text{ g}^{-1} \text{ mCi}^{-1} \text{ at 1 cm} \qquad (11.9)$$

$$= 4.42\,\bar{E} \text{ rad h}^{-1} \text{ mCi}^{-1} \text{ at 1 cm}$$

and the exposure rate from 1 mCi at 1 cm, for energies between 200 and 2000 KeV, expressed in roentgens

$$= 4.42\,\bar{E}/0.88$$

$$= 5\,\bar{E} \text{ R h}^{-1} \text{ mCi}^{-1} \text{ at 1 cm} \qquad (11.10)$$

The corresponding absorption dose rate in tissue, and the dose equivalent rate, can be calculated in rads and rems per hour respectively, using the relationships established on p. 196.

In SI units the exposure rate constant would be expressed as the exposure rate in air at 1 cm from a point source of 1 GBq of a particular nuclide, expressed in $\mathrm{C\,kg^{-1}\,h^{-1}}$.
From equation 11.9, the energy absorption rate in air per gigabecquerel

$$= \frac{(4.42 \times 10^{-5})\,\bar{E}\,10^9\,10^3}{(3.7 \times 10^7)}\ \mathrm{J\,h^{-1}\,kg^{-1}\,GBq^{-1}}\ \text{at 1 cm}$$

$$= 1.19\,\bar{E}\ \mathrm{Gy\,h^{-1}\,GBq^{-1}}\ \text{at 1 cm} \qquad (11.11)$$

From equation 11.10, the exposure rate from 1 GBq at 1 cm

$$= \frac{5\,\bar{E}\,10^9\,(2.58 \times 10^{-4})}{(3.7 \times 10^7)}$$

$$= 0.035\,\bar{E}\ \mathrm{C\,kg^{-1}\,h^{-1}\,GBq^{-1}}\ \text{at 1 cm} \qquad (11.12)$$

The corresponding absorption dose rate in tissue, and the dose-equivalent rate, can be calculated in grays and sieverts per hour respectively, using the relationship established in the previous section (p. 196).

In old units the exposure rate constant in $\mathrm{R\,h^{-1}\,mCi^{-1}}$ at 1 cm is approximately five times the mean γ-ray energy for energies between 0.08 and 3 MeV, and in SI units in $\mathrm{C\,kg^{-1}\,h^{-1}\,GBq^{-1}}$ at 1 cm is approximately 0.035 times the γ-ray energies. For lower

Table 11.5 *Exposure rate constants*

Nuclide	Principal γ- and X-ray energies (MeV)		Average γ-ray energy per disintegration (MeV)		Exposure rate constants: $\mathrm{R\,mCi^{-1}\,h^{-1}}$ at 1 cm		Exposure rate constants: $\mathrm{C\,kg^{-1}\,GBq^{-1}\,h^{-1}}$ at 1 cm	
^{125}I	0.027	(134%)	0.039		0.6		0.0042	
	0.035	(6.7%)						
^{99m}Tc	0.14	(88%)	0.126		0.77		0.00539	
^{123}I	0.028	(87%)	0.025	0.159	0.38	1.05	0.00266	0.0073
	0.16	(83%)	0.134		0.67		0.00469	
^{131}I	0.36	(83%)	0.384		2.2		0.0154	
	0.64	(6.9%)						
^{51}Cr	0.32	(9%)	0.03		0.16		0.00112	
^{113m}In	0.025	(24%)	0.006	0.260	0.1	1.4	0.0007	0.0098
	0.39	(65%)	0.254		1.3		0.0091	
^{59}Fe	1.10	(56%)	1.19		6.5		0.0455	
	1.29	(43%)						
^{24}Na	1.37	(100%)	4.12		18.4		0.129	
	2.75	(100%)						

γ-ray energies the absorption is greater, and therefore the exposure rate constant is greater than as calculated above. Values of the constant may be found in *The Radiochemical Manual* (Wilson, 1966) and some typical values are given in Table 11.5, in both units. It will be noticed that the value for ^{125}I is greater than given by equations 11.10 and 11.12.

If Γ is known, the γ-ray exposure rate due to any point source of radioactivity under given conditions can be calculated, and also the energy absorption rate in air and in tissue and the dose-equivalent rate due to that radiation exposure.

$$\text{Exposure} = \frac{\Gamma A e^{-\mu x} t}{d^2} \text{ R} \qquad (11.13)$$

where A = activity of source in mCi
$e^{-\mu x}$ = absorption in protective shielding
t = time of exposure in hours
d = distance from the source in cm

With a source other than a point source the self absorption, i.e. absorption in the source itself, must be taken into account. It is evident that for a given source the three variable factors which control exposure are time, distance and shielding, and these must be exploited to the best advantage.

For example, in handling a source the exposure may be reduced by using forceps or a remote-control device to increase the distance, or by using lead shielding between the source and the operator. It is essential that such devices are easy to manipulate, in order that their use does not result in long handling times which would offset the advantage gained. In some circumstances, speed of handling alone will keep exposure within acceptable limits.

It is always useful to have a rough idea of the radiation exposure. Some values of exposure rate which may be encountered in practice when handling vials and syringes containing radioactive solutions are given in Table 11.6. Exposure rates to hands when in contact with the surface of syringes and vials are given for these containers when they are unshielded and when they are shielded with appropriate thicknesses of lead. Exposure rates at 10 cm and 30 cm distances are also given for both shielded and unshielded sources; these represent, respectively, the exposure rates to the hands when short (10 cm) forceps are used, and to the whole body assuming a working distance of 30 cm. The exposure rates are given in R h^{-1} and C kg^{-1} h^{-1}; also given are the times for each exposure in which the worker would receive the MPD and the DEL (where the latter is different) for one working day, for the fingers or whole body as appropriate. It is obvious that the exposure rates at the surface of containers and at 10 cm are applicable to the finger dose, for which the MPD is 300 mrem (3 mSv) and the DEL is 2 mSv. The exposure rates at 30 cm are applicable to whole-body exposure, for which the MPD is 20 mrem (0.2 mSv) and the DEL is also 0.2 mSv. A better appreciation of radiation hazard is obtained if radiation exposures are expressed in this way.

γ-radiation absorbed dose due to internally administered radionuclides

For patients it is the radiation dose due to internal administration of radioactive material that is important. In this case it is important to know the distribution of the material within the body, and the rate of metabolism; if this information is available it is possible to determine the dose to the 'critical' organ (that is the organ which receives the highest dose) in relation to the maximum permissible level, and it is this dose which sets the limit on the amount of radioactivity which may be safely administered.

The γ-radiation absorbed dose in the body was originally estimated by using the specific γ-ray constant and a geometrical factor which allowed for the difference in absorption with various geometrical shapes.

In 1964 the American Society of Nuclear Medicine set up the Medical Internal Radiation Dose Committee (MIRD) with the objective of providing 'the best possible estimate of the absorbed dose to patients resulting from the diagnostic or therapeutic use of internally administered radiopharmaceuticals'. In 1968 the first MIRD pamphlet was published, entitled 'A scheme for absorbed-dose calculations for biologically-distributed radionuclides' (MIRD, 1968). The method makes use of the concept of an absorbed fraction or a specific absorbed fraction. It starts with the hypothesis that for a uniform distribution of a radionuclide in an infinite, homogeneous absorbing material, the energy absorbed per gram is in equilibrium with the energy emitted per gram, and the equilibrium absorbed dose is given by

$$D \text{ equil} = \widetilde{C}\, \Sigma_i\, \Delta_i \text{ rad} \qquad (11.14)$$

where $\widetilde{C}$ = integrated concentration of radioactivity over its whole life, in μCi h g^{-1}

Table 11.6 *Exposure rates due to the γ-radiation (expressed in R hour^{-1} and C kg^{-1} hour^{-1} respectively) from 1 mCi and 1 GBq of nuclides of different energies, under various conditions*

Nuclide	Main γ-ray energy (MeV)	Volume of solution and type of container	In contact: Exposure rate[a] A	In contact: Exposure rate[a] B	In contact: Time (min) to receive MPD[b]	In contact: Time (min) to receive DEL[c]	At 10 cm distance: Exposure rate[a] C	At 10 cm distance: Exposure rate[a] D	At 10 cm distance: Time (h) to receive MPD[b]	At 10 cm distance: Time (h) to receive DEL[c]	At 30 cm distance: Exposure rate[a] C	At 30 cm distance: Exposure rate[a] D	At 30 cm distance: Time (h) to receive MPD[d]	At 30 cm distance: Time (h) to receive DEL[d]	In contact with screening: Screen (mm Pb)	In contact with screening: Exposure rate[a] C	In contact with screening: Exposure rate[a] D	In contact with screening: Time (h) to receive MPD[b]	In contact with screening: Time (h) to receive DEL[c]
^{125}I	0.027	1 ml in glass vial	1.84	12.9	10	0.25	18	129	17	0.42	1.8	12.9	10	0.25	0.1 (or 1 cm Al)	20	140	15	0.38
^{99m}Tc	0.14	10 ml in glass vaccine bottle	0.42	2.94	43	1.06	4.2	28	70	1.7	0.42	2.8	48	1.25	1.0	28	196	21	0.28
		1 ml in disposable syringe	2.64	18.4	6.8	0.17	26	184	11	0.3	2.6	18.4	15	0.38	1.0 2.0	179 12	1253 84	1.7 24	0.043 0.64
^{131}I	0.36	1 ml in glass vial	2.28	15.9	7.9	0.19	23	160	13	0.3	2.3	16.0	12.5	0.3	13.0	47	329	6.4	0.16

[a]Exposure rates are given in R hour^{-1} mCi^{-1} (A), mC kg^{-1} hour^{-1} GBq^{-1} (B), mR hour^{-1} mCi^{-1} (C) and μC kg^{-1} hour^{-1} GBq^{-1} (D).
Times are also given in which the MPD for 1 working day would be received from 1 mCi and the DEL from 1 GBq:
[b]MPD to hands for 1 working day = 300 mrem (3 mSv);
[c]DEL for skin for 1 working day = 2 mSv (200 mrem);
[d]MPD and DEL for whole body (WB) for 1 working day = 200 mrem (0.2 mSv).

and

$$\Delta_i = 2.13\, n_i\, \overline{E}_i \text{ g-rad}/\mu\text{Ci h} \tag{11.15}$$

where $\overline{E}_i$ = energy emitted, in MeV, per μCi h in the form of *i*th-type radiation (see derivation of equation 11.19)

The expression for D equil (equation 11.14) takes into account the fact that the radionuclide may emit several, m, γ-rays of mean energies $\overline{E}_1\ \overline{E}_2 \ldots \overline{E}_i \ldots \overline{E}_m$ in the proportions $n_1\ n_2 \ldots n_i \ldots n_m$. The term $n_i\overline{E}_i$ is a general one, and the summation sign $\Sigma_i\, \Delta_i$ signifies the summation of the energies emitted by the several γ-rays per disintegration, that is the total energy emitted.

In terms of SI units

$$D \text{ equil} = \widetilde{C}\, \Sigma_i\, \Delta_i \text{ Gy}$$

where $\widetilde{C}$ is in Bq h g^{-1}
and

$$\Delta_i = (5.77 \times 10^{-7}) n_i\, \overline{E}_i \text{ g-Gy/Bq h} \tag{11.16}$$

where $\overline{E}_i$ is in MeV

The equilibrium absorbed dose is easily calculable from the above, provided that the distribution of the radioactivity is known and also its rate of turnover. The concept is then that there is a source region which contains the radioactivity, and a target region which absorbs the radiation; part or the whole of one region may be part or the whole of the other. A specific fraction of the equilibrium dose, as calculated for the source region, will be absorbed in the target region. This is expressed in symbols as

$$\widetilde{D}\,(r_1 \leftarrow r_2) = \widetilde{A}_2\ \Sigma_i\ \Delta_i\, \phi\,(r_1 \leftarrow r_2) \text{ rad} \tag{11.17}$$

which means: the mean radiation dose received in the target region (r_1) due to the radioactivity in the source region (r_2) is equal to the integrated activity over its whole life, of the activity ($\widetilde{A}_2$) in the source region, multiplied by the sum of the energies emitted per μCi h for each type of radiation, multiplied by the specific absorbed fraction for that type of radiation. The main difficulty is in the calculation of the specific absorbed fraction and this has been done using Monte Carlo techniques. For non-penetrating radiation, by definition, only an insignificant amount of energy is absorbed outside a source volume, and the radiation dose in this case is considered in the next section. For penetrating radiation, by definition, a significant amount of energy is absorbed outside the source volume. There are MIRD tables now available of the quantity $\Sigma_i \Delta_i \phi (r_1 \leftarrow r_2)$, denoted as $S (r_1 \leftarrow r_2)$, for many radionuclides and source–target configurations commonly encountered in nuclear medicine (MIRD, 1975). The cumulative activity $\widetilde{A}$ can be calculated from the biological data. When calculating the radiation dose to a given organ it is necessary to sum the doses to the organ from all source organs for which $\widetilde{A}$ is significant.

β-radiation absorbed dose

It will be seen from Table 11.1 (maximum range of β-particles) that β-radiation up to 0.35 MeV will be completely absorbed in 1 mm of polythene. It follows that when radioactive solutions are contained in a plastic, or glass, vial or syringe, any β-radiation of energy less than 0.35 MeV will be completely absorbed, and therefore there is no hazard from external radiation. The β-radiation of highest energy normally encountered in practice is the 1.69 MeV β-radiation from ^{32}P, and Table 11.1 shows that even this is easily absorbed by using a 1 mm lead shield, although it should be noted that the process of absorption of high-energy β-radiation involves the production of γ-radiation known as bremsstrahlung. The hazards from β-emitters are those which might arise when sources are spilt, or from skin contamination, ingestion or inhalation. The radiation dose from β-radiation, by deposition of radioactive material on the skin, or in the body, may be calculated as follows.

Since their range in tissue is very short, the β-rays are completely absorbed very close to the source. It may be taken, therefore, as an approximation, that the total energy is absorbed in the volume of distribution of the source.

The energy given off per millicurie is $(3.7 \times 10^7) \bar{E}_\beta (1.602 \times 10^{-13})$ J per second, where $\bar{E}_\beta$ is the mean energy of the β-radiation expressed in MeV.

With a concentration of 1 mCi deposited per gram of tissue,

$$\text{Energy absorbed} = \frac{(3.7 \times 10^7)\bar{E}_\beta (1.602 \times 10^{-13})}{10^{-5}}$$

rad per second/mCi per g tissue

$$= 0.59\, \bar{E}_\beta \text{ g-rad/mCi s}$$

$$= 2.13\, \bar{E}_\beta \text{ g-rad}/\mu\text{Ci h} \tag{11.18}$$

If there are i types of β-radiation of energy $\bar{E}_i$ which occur in the proportion n_i then the mean β-ray energy will be given by

$$\bar{E}_\beta = \Sigma_i\, n_i\, \bar{E}_i \tag{11.19}$$

and

$$\text{energy absorbed} = 2.13\, \Sigma_i\, n_i\, \bar{E}_i \text{ g-rad}/\mu\text{Ci h}$$

which is the equilibrium absorbed dose (D equil) of equation 11.15, for a concentration of 1 μCi g^{-1}.

In terms of SI units

$$\text{energy absorbed} = (3.6 \times 10^6)\, \Sigma_i\, n_i\, \bar{E}_i \text{ g-Gy/Bq h} \tag{11.20}$$

when $\bar{E}$ is in joules
or

$$\text{energy absorbed} = (5.77 \times 10^{-7})\, \Sigma_i\, n_i\, \bar{E}_i \text{ g-Gy/Bq h} \tag{11.21}$$

when $\bar{E}$ is in MeV

When considering skin contamination it may be assumed that one-half of the β-ray energy is absorbed in the superficial layers of the skin, in a depth equal to the average range of the β-radiation, which is approximately one-third of the maximum range. For example, suppose 0.01 ml (which is one drop from a syringe with a No. 1 needle) of a solution of ^{32}P of concentration 1 mCi ml^{-1} (which is encountered when ^{32}P is used therapeutically) is dropped on to the skin, and the drop, containing 10 μCi, spreads over an area 1 cm in diameter. The maximum β-ray energy of ^{32}P is 1.71 MeV, and the maximum range is 8.2 mm in tissue. The average range is about 2.7 mm.

Surface contamination = 10 μCi cm^{-2} approximately

Volume of tissue involved = surface area $\times$ average range

$$= \Pi\, 0.5^2\, 0.27 = 0.2 \text{ cm}^3$$

$$\text{Concentration of } ^{32}\text{P in tissue} = \frac{10}{0.2} = 50\ \mu\text{Ci cm}^{-3}$$

$$= 50\ \mu\text{Ci g}^{-1}$$

(since the density of tissue $\approx$ 1 g cm^{-3})

Mean β-ray energy of ^{32}P = 0.6 MeV

From equation 11.18,

$$\text{Radiation dose rate} = \tfrac{1}{2}\ 2.13\ 0.6\ 50 \text{ rad hour}^{-1}$$
$$= 32 \text{ rad hour}^{-1}$$

In SI units

$$\text{Concentration of } ^{32}\text{P in tissue} = 50\,(3.7 \times 10^4) \text{ Bq cm}^{-3}$$
$$= 1.85 \times 10^6 \text{ Bq cm}^{-3}$$

From equation 11.21,

$$\text{Radiation dose rate} = \tfrac{1}{2}(5.77 \times 10^{-7})0.6(1.85 \times 10^6)$$
$$= 0.32 \text{ Gy hour}^{-1}$$

For solutions of technetium-99m of concentration 1 mCi ml^{-1}, which are in common use, the radiation dose due to a similar drop on the skin is of the same order. The mean β-ray energy, mainly from internal conversion electrons, is 0.123 MeV, and occurs in 12% of disintegrations. The mean range is 0.02 cm.

$$\Sigma n_i E_i = 0.12 \times 0.123 = 0.0143 \text{ MeV}$$

$$\text{Volume of tissue involved} = (\Pi/4)0.02 = 0.0158 \text{ cm}^3$$

$$\text{Concentration of } ^{99\text{m}}\text{Tc in tissue} = 10/0.0158$$
$$= 633\ \mu\text{Ci cm}^{-3}$$

$$\text{Radiation dose rate} = \tfrac{1}{2} \times 2.13 \times 0.0143 \times 633$$
$$= 9.7 \text{ rad hour}^{-1}$$

In SI units

$$\text{Concentration of } ^{99\text{m}}\text{Tc in tissue} = 633(3.7 \times 10^4) \text{ Bq cm}^{-3}$$
$$= 2.33 \times 10^7 \text{ Bq cm}^{-3}$$

$$\text{Radiation dose rate} = \tfrac{1}{2}(5.77 \times 10^{-7}) \times 0.0143 \times (2.33 \times 10^7)$$
$$= 0.1 \text{ Gy hour}^{-1}$$

These are very high dose-rates. An important rule which prevents accidental skin contamination is to wear gloves when handling any radioactive solution of radioactive concentration greater than 0.1 μCi ml^{-1} (3.7 kBq ml^{-1}).

The maximum permissible level for skin contamination, as recommended in the Code of Practice (Table 11.7) is 10^{-4} μCi

cm^{-2} (3.7 Bq cm^{-2}) (which gives a radiation dose-rate of about 1 mrad per hour (10 μGy per hour)), averaged over an area of 100 cm^2, except for the hands where it is averaged over the area of the whole hand, taken as 300 cm^2, to give a maximum permissible level of 3×10^{-2} μCi (1.1 kBq) per hand. The MPD to the hands for occupationally-exposed persons is 75 rems (0.75 Sv) per year (ICRP, 1965), that is 1.4 rems (14 mSv) per week and 9 mrems (0.09 mSv) per hour, for continuous exposure. The latest ICRP recommendations (ICRP, 1977*b*), do not give a DEL specifically for the hands, but give a DEL of 500 mSv per year for skin, that is 10 mSv per week, and 0.06 mSv per hour; these values are 33% lower than the MPD values. The maximum permissible level of contamination when applied to the hands, assuming it to be continuous and uniform over the whole hand, would give a radiation dose equal to about one-tenth of the MPD and DEL levels, and allows a safety factor if the contamination were not uniform but concentrated in a small area.

Legal requirements for the UK

Council Directive of 1 June 1976 (European Communities)
The above directive laying down basic safety standards was referred to in Chapter 5 with respect to regulations concerning

Table 11.7 *Working limits for surface contamination*

Category	Surface	Derived working limit	
		μCi cm^{-2}	Bq cm^{-2}
A	Surfaces of the interiors and contents of glove boxes and fume cupboards	The minimum that is reasonably practicable	
B	Surfaces of active areas and of plant, apparatus, equipment (including personal protective equipment), materials and articles within active areas other than those of category A	All radionuclides except tritium and α-emitters[a]	
		10^{-3}	37
C	Surfaces of the body	10^{-4}	3.7
D	All other surfaces, e.g. inactive areas, personal clothing, hospital bedding	10^{-4}	3.7

From DHSS (1972).
[a]These figures are not applicable to tritium. It is difficult to measure tritium contamination on surfaces, and where it is considered necessary control should be by urine analysis.

administration of radiopharmaceuticals. The requirements of the directive concerning radiation dose limitation will now be considered. Since it preceded ICRP Publication 26 (referred to earlier in this chapter), the directive adopted the MPD values in ICRP Publication 9. At the time of going to press, a new EC directive has been drafted and is about to be issued; it is understood that this takes into account the terms and values recommended in ICRP Publication 26, as set out in Table 11.3, and the gradual introduction of SI units. The implementation date of the directive has been delayed, and it is now expected to be 1 July 1980.

The directive applies to the production, processing, handling, use, holding, storage, transport and disposal of natural and artificial radioactive substances and to any other activity which involves a hazard arising from ionising radiation. It stipulates the limitation of radiation doses for controllable exposure, and also limits for intake and for concentration of radionuclides in air. It lays down fundamental principles governing the health surveillance of exposed workers, including clarification and demarcation of areas, classification of exposed workers, assessment of exposure and medical surveillance of exposed workers.

Ionising radiations regulations in the UK

In the UK, the Health and Safety at Work etc. Act became law in 1974, and a body known as the Health and Safety Council (HSC) has been formed under the Department of Employment. the HSC is responsible for the production of legislative regulations, as required by the EC directive, to cover all aspects of the handling and use of radioactive materials and ionising radiations, except the administration of radiopharmaceuticals which is covered under the Medicines Act, and has been discussed in Chapter 5. The HSC has issued a consultative document entitled *Ionising Radiations: Proposals for Provisions on Radiological Protection* (HMSO, 1978). They intend to publish, in 1979, draft regulations, approved code, and guidance notes, for the proposed legislative document. The draft will be circulated for three months, and the final document, as presented to Parliament, is expected to be published in late 1979 for implementation by 1 July 1980. All workers exposed to ionising radiations must be familiar with these regulations. The Ionising Radiations (Sealed Sources) Regulations 1969 and The Ionising Radiations (Unsealed Radioactive Substances) Regulations 1968 will continue to be in force until the new regulations come into operation, when the former will be revoked. The current regulations require all users of radioactive sources to be registered, and to obtain authorisation before holding stocks of, or disposing of, radioactive materials. They require that records are kept, and are available for inspection by representatives of the Department of the Environment.

Code of Practice and local rules

In the UK there is a *Code of Practice for the Protection of Persons against Ionising Radiations arising from Medical and Dental Use* (DHSS, 1972). It does not have statutory force, but the DHSS has issued a directive to the institutions concerned for its implementation. The *Code* is being revised by the National Radiological Protection Board (NRPB) to take account of the EC Directive and the forthcoming HSE regulations. There is also a *Code of Practice for the Protection of Persons Exposed to Ionising Radiations in Research and Teaching* (DHSS, 1968), which has been reprinted without any change of content but is now entitled *Guidance* instead of *Code of Practice.*

The *Code* requires that all DHSS centres draw up local rules to conform with the *Code*. All workers must be familiar with the local rules applying to all the departments in which they work. A typical set of local rules is given in the appendix to this chapter; they are concerned with radiological protection and do not include rules to be observed with regard to maintaining pharmaceutical purity of radiopharmaceuticals. It should be noted that the rules with respect to the disposal of radioactive waste (Appendix, p. 215) and the records of radioactive materials (Appendix, p. 217) are mandatory.

Appendix. Typical set of local rules

Introduction

The Department is divided into:

(*a*) A 'hot' area which comprises:

- (i) A 'hot' dispensing and radiochemical laboratory for the handling of doses or samples greater than 1 mCi. The ^{99m}Tc and ^{113}In generators are kept permanently in this room.
- (ii) A high-activity measurement room for activities greater than 1 mCi.

(iii) A room containing the radioactive store and the sluice for disposal of radioactive waste.

(*b*) A low-level dispensing laboratory for handling doses or samples less than 1 mCi.

(*c*) A sample counting laboratory.

(*d*) Five rooms in which measurements are carried out on patients.

The two dispensing laboratories and the sluice constitute the active areas and all dispensing of radioactive materials must be carried out in the laboratory appropriate for the activity level.

No manipulations of radioactive material must be carried out elsewhere in the department, with the following exceptions:

(*a*) The administration of oral or intravenous therapy doses, which is done in the high-activity measurement room.

(*b*) The administration of oral or intravenous tracer doses, which is done in the appropriate patient room.

Cleaning, other than floors, must not be carried out by domestic staff in the 'hot' dispensing and radiochemical laboratory or in the radioactive store room without prior permission, in every case, from the Radiological Safety Officer.

Rules for handling unsealed sources

There are three main hazards in handling unsealed sources of radioactivity, these are:

(1) Deposition of isotopes in the body.

(2) Skin contamination and spread of contamination.

(3) Effects of external β- and γ-radiation.

The rules are accordingly grouped into three parts, each based on controlling one of the hazards.

1. To avoid deposition of isotopes in the body

These rules apply to all levels of radioactivity.

(i) Laboratory coats must always be worn in the laboratories.

(ii) No eating, drinking, smoking, etc., in either the 'hot area' or the low-level dispensing laboratory.

(iii) Gloves must be worn for all procedures involving solutions with radioactive concentration greater than 0.1 μCi ml^{-1}, and larger volumes of lower concentration but total activity greater than 10 μCi.

(iv) Hands must be monitored immediately after handling any activity greater than 1 mCi, and also before going home and going to meals. They must be checked after removing the gloves. If the check shows a level of activity greater than the stipulated level, the hands must be thoroughly re-washed, and if the activity persists the Radiological Safety Officer must be informed.

(v) All radioactive sources of concentration greater than 0.01 μCi ml^{-1} or total content greater than 1 μCi must be clearly labelled, stating the isotope, activity, date and volume. This must be done before, or immediately after, preparation.

(vi) Pipetting must always be carried out by remote control, *never* by mouth.

2. To avoid skin contamination and spread of contamination
The 'hot' dispensing laboratory and the low-level dispensing laboratory must be strictly segregated.

(i) *Work in hot laboratory*, i.e. all activities greater than 1 mCi.

Disposable gloves must always be worn when actually handling the activity. Gloves should not be worn outside the hot laboratory. After use, gloves should be removed, using the surgical technique, and placed in the radioactive bin.

The possibility of transferring activity to the skin, or any inactive region or object, should always be kept in mind, and meticulous care must be exercised. For example, in the event of any drips or splashes getting on the hands, the gloves should be immediately washed off, or swabbed dry, before proceeding. They should then be removed as soon as possible afterwards.

All operations must be carried out over a drip tray which should be covered with absorbent paper.

Radioactive iodine must be handled and dispensed in a fume cupboard with adequate ventilation.

Glassware, polythene-ware, syringes, pipettes, etc. Wherever it is possible, disposable containers and instruments should be used. Glassware and polythene-ware which is not disposable is marked according to the isotope and activity; the correct items should be used.

Syringes are all disposable. Contaminated syringes should, however, be rinsed out *before* the needle is removed and placed in the appropriate 'active box' and the syringe placed in the radioactive bin. (If a procedure is being carried out which involves the use of many syringes, a plastic bag should be at hand, and the syringes and other contaminated items placed in it.)

Pipettes are marked according to the isotope and activity, and the correct pipette should be used. They must not be left to drip except over a container. Pipettes must first be rinsed, either directly in the sink (if this is empty) or placed in a large beaker (appropriate grade of activity). They must *not* be left on the bench.

No contaminated material of any description must be

left lying about on the benches or draining board. If it is not possible to clear up straight away, it must be placed on the shelves provided for the purpose. Levels of activity must be segregated. Levels should not be mixed while washing up.

All other tools, e.g. bottle opener, which have been used must be checked for contamination before being put away.

Equipment used in the hot laboratory must not be taken for use outside.

(ii) *Work in low-level dispensing laboratories*, i.e. activities less than 1 mCi.

While the hazard is much less than in handling high activities, there is still need for great care to avoid cross contamination which can invalidate results.

Disposable gloves must be worn for all procedures involving activities greater than 0.1 μCi ml^{-1}. The possibility of transferring activity to the skin or any inactive region or object should always be kept in mind, and sound commonsense used to avoid this.

All operations must be carried out over a drip tray.

Glassware, syringes etc. Disposable ware should be used whenever possible. All contaminated syringes should be rinsed out *before* the needle is removed. Needles may then be removed and placed in the appropriate box and the syringe placed in the radioactive bin. Other contaminated ware should be rinsed out straight away if not disposable.

No contaminated material must be left lying about on benches or draining boards.

(iii) *Monitoring*

The benches in the tracer dispensing laboratory and the hot laboratory must be monitored at the end of every working week. Permissible level of contamination is 10^{-3} μCi cm^{-2} (i.e. 37 disintegrations cm^{-2} per second) averaged over an area not greater than 300 cm^2. The results must be recorded.

If any spillage of radioactive material occurs, in either dispensing laboratory, it is the duty of the person involved to deal with the situation immediately. Personnel contamination, and/or invalidation of important clinical results may occur if there is lack of self-discipline in this respect.

3. To avoid effects of external γ- and β-radiation

(i) *γ-radiation*

(*a*) Microcurie sources. These constitute no hazard as long as reasonable care is used. These sources may be picked up by hand but should not be handled for prolonged periods of time.

(*b*) Millicurie sources. These constitute a potential hazard and the following precautions should be taken:
   (i) At all times when the source is not being used, store in a lead pot of suitable thickness.
   (ii) Transport in a suitable lead pot or long-handled container.
   (iii) Do not pick up by hand but use tongs or forceps.
   (iv) Carry out all manipulations, i.e. when the source is outside its lead pot, as quickly as possible, and do not get nearer to the source than is absolutely necessary.

(ii) *β-radiation*
The only β-emitter currently used of which the β-rays are sufficiently energetic to penetrate the glass walls of bottles or syringes is ^{32}P. This should be handled in the container provided and a 0.5 mm lead shield used for the syringe.

Emergency procedures

Staff must be fully conversant with their duties in the event of a radiation accident involving personal injury, a spill of radioactivity, or a fire.

1. Accident involving personal injury
In the event of personal injury, the treatment of the injury must take precedence, even with contaminated persons. It may, however, be possible to 'contain' the contamination by taking any such persons to the same area and immediately alerting the medical and nursing staff to the problem.

The treatment of *serious* injuries must take precedence over all other considerations. Send the injured person under escort to the casualty department and warn them of his arrival. Inform the Safety Medical Officer, Radiological Protection Adviser and Radiological Safety Officer.

Minor injuries should be treated at, or near, the scene of the incident. Wash any wound under a tap with copious quantities of water and encourage bleeding. If the wound is on the face, take care not to contaminate the eyes, mouth or nostrils.

Wash the wound with soap and water and apply a first-aid dressing.

The injured area should be monitored to establish the level of residual activity, if any.

2. Major spills, i.e. those involving millicurie amounts

Spills of millicurie amounts are serious, particularly if personnel are involved. These large quantities are generally used in therapeutic doses. Millicurie amounts of short-lived isotopes are also used in many tracer investigations; these are less hazardous but the procedure given below should be adopted. The following action should be taken, using the 'Decontamination Kit':

(*a*) Assistance must be called, and the head of the department and the Radiological Safety Officer informed at once.

(*b*) The affected area must be screened off. Anyone entering this area must wear overshoes and gloves, both of which must be removed on leaving the area and placed in the bag provided.

(*c*) All non-contaminated persons should be removed from the area.

(*d*) All contaminated non-injured persons should be kept in a separate screened off area; all contaminated clothing must be removed and placed in the bag provided. If the spill is on the skin, the area should be flushed thoroughly with tap water, taking great care not to spread the contamination, particularly to the eyes. The skin should be monitored; decontamination measures should aim at getting the activity down to 10^{-4} μCi cm^{-2} averaged over 100 cm^2.

(*e*) The actual material spilt must be mopped up with absorbent paper, which should be put in the bag provided.

(*f*) The contaminated surface must be washed until the activity is down to the maximum permissible level (10^{-3} μCi cm^{-2} averaged over 100 cm^2 for active areas). If this cannot be achieved the area must be covered over with polythene sheeting.

3. Minor spills, i.e. those involving microcurie amounts

These spills are not serious but require careful handling to avoid spreading contamination. The following procedures should be adopted, using the 'Decontamination Kit':

(*a*) Gloves must be put on before dealing with the spill.

(*b*) If personnel are involved any contaminated clothing must be removed immediately and put in a suitable container for monitoring.

If any of the radioactive material is on the skin, the area should be flushed thoroughly with tap water (taking care to avoid the spread of contamination) and then washed with soap and water.

(*c*) The spill should be mopped up with absorbent paper, and the paper placed in the bag provided.

(*d*) The contaminated area must be monitored before it is put back into use.

4. Fire hazard
In the event of fire, personnel should follow the hospital fire drill, unless the outbreak is very limited. The head of department, Custodian of Unsealed Sources, and the Radiological Safety Officer will, if possible, see that the doors of the radioactive store and the radiopharmaceutical laboratory are closed. If there is time, any radioactive sources greater than 1 mCi will be returned to one of those rooms.

Disposal of radioactive waste

Liquid waste
The hospital is permitted to dispose of up to a sum total of *500 mCi* of all radionuclides in any one calendar month. The Department of the Environment, however, demands that records are kept of all waste disposal. The disposal of all liquid waste of activity greater than 100 μCi must be entered in the disposal book, recording the date, nuclide and approximate activity.

All activities greater than 100 μCi should be disposed of directly into the sluice and, of course, also recorded. Activities of up to a total of 100 μCi in any one day may be disposed of down any designated sink.

Solid waste
The regulations for solid waste are much more stringent than for liquid waste, the hospital being permitted to dispose of not more than the sum total of 3 mCi of all radionuclides in any one week with the exception of radioiodine for which it has a special authorisation to dispose of up to 12 mCi as solid waste during the same period.

Miscellaneous solid waste, comprising items of activity less than about 10 μCi, may be placed in the General Radioactive Bin. This bin must be emptied regularly, as necessary, at intervals not exceeding one week; its contents must be monitored and recorded before disposal. Items of solid waste known to contain activity greater than about 10 μCi must be labelled (after assaying if necessary), recorded separately, and placed in the Specific-Item Radioactive Bin.

All solid waste must be sent direct to the incinerator for disposal according to the Current Regulations.

Excreta

Except when required for radioactivity tests, excreta from patients should be disposed of to the sewer, preferably by the patient using the toilet directly. However, records should be kept of the approximate amount of radioactivity excreted, and the place of disposal. The activity of the excreta may be estimated as stated in the procedure books.

Drains

The Radiological Safety Officer should be informed if it is necessary to make repairs to the drains serving the main sluice in the radioisotope department.

Duties of radiological safety officer

(i) To see that all instructions in the Code of Practice and Local Rules are observed in the department for which the officer is responsible.

(ii) To make sure that the personnel monitoring devices are in good working condition and used where indicated.

(iii) To instruct, in collaboration with the head of department and other senior staff, personnel in safe working practices.

(iv) To establish and maintain operational procedures so that the radiation exposure of each worker is kept as far below the maximum permissible level as is practicable.

(v) To ensure in collaboration with the head of the department that there is adequate protection to cover all changes in procedure and any new procedures. Dummy runs should be carried out if necessary.

(vi) To report to the head of department, when it is suspected that a hazard exists.

(vii) To report to the head of department any repeated breaking of the protection rules by members of the staff.

(viii) To monitor personnel when required.

(ix) To check that benches and sink outflows are monitored at weekly intervals, and that the checks are recorded.

(x) To deal with radioactive spills in the Radioisotope Department and on the wards. To advise on the handling of spills in any other department.

(xi) To report *in writing* via the Head of the Department to the Radiological Protection Adviser:

- (*a*) Any new procedure and/or isotopes being used.
- (*b*) Any deterioration in the state of protection in the department including details of any equipment required for protection.

(xii) To report *in writing* to the Radiological Protection Adviser as soon as possible any accidents involving major spills, and the steps taken to avoid repetition.

Duties of the Custodian of Unsealed Radioactive Sources
Radioactive sources are stored in two main areas:

(i) In the 'hot' area store room the sources are of low activity and are stored in a steel safe. The sources comprise:
    (*a*) Activities of the order of a few millicuries of various radionuclides in use for tracer investigations.
    (*b*) Occasional therapeutic doses of iodine-131, gold-198, and phosphorus-32 which are kept overnight in the safe.

(ii) In the 'hot' area radiochemical laboratory the sources are the molybdenum-technetium-99m generator, and the tin–indium-113m generator. These are the highest activity sources in the department.

In addition, very low activities of radiopharmaceuticals that have to be stored at low temperatures, are kept in the refrigerator and the deep freezer.

In view of the fact that the activities are low, and are in constant use, except for the overnight storage of therapeutic doses, the stores may be handled as an auxiliary store. Therefore, it is not necessary to record each movement of every source within the department.

The Custodian of Unsealed Radioactive Sources will be responsible for ensuring that the following duties are carried out by the appointed technician:

(i) To receive all the sources coming into the department, and check the activity of each source in the standard ionisation chamber wherever possible. For low-activity γ-ray emitters which cannot be measured in the standard ionisation chamber, i.e. [^{58}Co] vitamin B12, an alternative method of checking must be used. For low-energy β-emitters it is not possible to check the activity without opening the container. The nominal activity stated on the label is, therefore, accepted as correct. The receipt of each source and its measurement must be recorded in the appropriate book. All sources must be put either in the safe or the refrigerator, or issued to the appropriate department on the day of arrival.

(ii) To issue all sources for therapeutic doses.

(iii) To check the contents of the safe regularly each week and to adjust the record for amounts used, for radioactive decay, and for sources disposed of.

(iv) To record the activity of all sources issued to other departments, excluding those sources which are unopened in the Radioisotope Department (these, if delivered to the Radioisotope Department, will be recorded in the diary).

(v) To ensure that a record is kept of all radionuclides coming into the hospital. This record must show quite clearly, for each department involved, the total quantity of each radionuclide received.

(vi) To ensure that all containers in the stores are clearly labelled, indicating the isotope, activity, date to which activity relates, also chemical form and radioactive concentration if relevant.

References

DHSS (1968). *Code of Practice for the Protection of Persons Exposed to Ionising Radiations in Teaching and Research.* London: HMSO.

DHSS (1972). *Code of Practice for the Protection of Persons against Ionising Radiations arising from Medical and Dental Use.* London: HMSO.

EC Council Directive (1976). Council Directive of 1 June 1976 laying down the revised basic safety standards for the health protection of the general public and workers against the dangers of ionising radiation. *Official Journal of the European Communities*, **19**, no. L187.

HMSO (1968). *The Ionising Radiations (Unsealed Radioactive Substances) Regulations.* London: HMSO.

HMSO (1969). *The Ionising Radiations (Sealed Sources) Regulations).* London: HMSO.

HMSO (1978). *Ionising Radiations: Proposals for Provisions on Radiological Protection.* London: HMSO.

ICRP (1959). *Recommendations of the International Committees on Radiological Protection: Report of Committee II on Permissible Doses for Internal Radiation.* ICRP Publication 2. Oxford: Pergamon Press.

ICRP (1964). *Recommendations of the International Commission on Radiological Protection.* ICRP Publication 6. Oxford: Pergamon Press.

ICRP (1965). *Recommendations of the International Commission on Radiological Protection.* ICRP Publication 9. Oxford: Pergamon Press.

ICRP (1971). *Protection of the Patient in Radionuclidic Investigations.* ICRP Publication 17. Oxford: Pergamon Press.

ICRP (1977*a*). *The Handling, Storage, Use and Disposal of Unsealed Radionuclides in Hospitals and Medical Research Establishments.* ICRP Publication 25. Oxford: Pergamon Press.

ICRP (1977*b*). *Recommendations of the International Commission on Radiological Protection.* ICRP Publication 26. Oxford: Pergamon Press.

ICRP (1979). *Limits for Intakes of Radionuclides by Workers*, vol. 1. ICRP Publication 30. Oxford: Pergamon Press (in preparation).

MIRD (1968). A scheme for absorbed-dose calculations for biologically distributed radionuclides. *J. Nucl. Med.*, suppl. 1, 7–14.

MIRD (1975). *Radionuclide Decay Schemes and Nuclear Parameters for use in Radiation-dose Estimation.* nm/mird pamphlet 10. New York: The Society of Nuclear Medicine.

NBS (1956/8). *Energy Loss and Range of Electrons and Positrons.* National Bureau of Standards Circular 577 and Supplement. Washington, DC: US Government Printing Office.

NBS (1957). *X-ray Attenuation Coefficients from 10keV to 100 MeV.* National Bureau of Standards Circular 583. Washington, DC: National Bureau of Standards.

Wilson, B.J. (1966). *The Radiochemical Manual*, 2nd edn. Amersham: The Radiochemical Centre.

Glossary of terms and units

Words that are italicised have separate entries.

absorbed dose	Energy imparted by *ionising radiations* to unit mass of matter. The old unit of absorbed dose is the *rad*. The new SI unit is the *gray*.
activity (of a radioactive source)	The number of disintegrations taking place per unit time. The old unit of activity is the *curie*. The new SI unit is the *becquerel*.
alpha-particle (α-particle)	A positively charged particle emitted in the radioactive decay of some nuclei, e.g. radium. Identical with the *nucleus* of the helium-4 atom.
annihilation radiation	Two *photons* of *gamma radiation* produced when a *positron* combines with an *electron*. Each photon is of energy 0.51 MeV, and they are emitted in opposite directions.
atom	The smallest amount of an element which has the properties of that element. The atom consists of a central *nucleus* around which *electrons* move in orbits.
atomic number of an element (Z)	The numerical place occupied by the element in the Periodic Table. It is equal to the number of *protons* in the *nucleus* of the *atom*. In the uncharged atom this is also equal to the number of *electrons*, and therefore determines the chemical properties of the element.
becquerel (Bq)	The *SI unit* of *activity* (of a radioactive source). One becquerel is the activity of a source in which the rate of disintegration is 1 per second.
beta-particle (β-particle)	An *electron* given off during the *radioactive decay* of *nuclei*.
characteristic X-radiation	Electromagnetic radiation given off when an atom in an excited state reverts to its normal energy state. The excitation may be caused by the removal of one of the orbital *electrons*, as for example in *electron capture*.
coulomb per kilogram ($C\ kg^{-1}$)	The *SI* unit of *exposure*.
curie (Ci)	The old unit of *activity*. One curie is the activity of a source in which the rate of disintegration is 3.7×10^{10} per second, i.e. 3.7×10^{10} Bq.
decay constant (λ)	The proportion of *nuclei* in a *radioactive* source which *disintegrate* in unit time ($dN/dt = \lambda N$).
disintegration	A spontaneous process in which the *nucleus* of an atom changes its form or its energy state, by emitting either particulate or electromagnetic radiation, or by *electron capture*.
dose equivalent	The *absorbed dose* multiplied by factors to allow for the different biological effect produced, for equal energy absorption, by different types of radiation, as well as other modifying effects. The old unit of dose equivalent is the *rem*. The *SI unit* is the *sievert*.
dose equivalent limit (DEL)	The numerical values recommended by the International Commission on Radiological Protection to be the controlling limits of radiation dose which should not be exceeded by radiation workers or by any maximally exposed group of the general public. The DEL supersede the MPD (maximum permissible dose).
electron	A fundamental particle of mass 9.109×10^{-31} kg ($0.000548\ m_u$) and having one unit of negative charge (1.602×10^{-19} C). A common constituent of all *atoms*.
electron capture	A mode of *radioactive disintegration* whereby the *nucleus* of the *atom* captures one of the orbital *electrons*, usually from the inner, K, shell, and leaves the atom in an excited state. The atom reverts to its ground state by emitting *characteristic X-radiation*.
electron-volt (eV)	A measure of energy of a particle or electromagnetic radiation. The kinetic energy acquired by an electron when it is accelerated across an electric potential of 1 volt. 1 eV $\approx 1.602 \times 10^{-19}$ J. The joule (J) is the *SI unit* of energy.

exposure — A measure of radiation based on its *ionising* properties; it is expressed as the charge of the *ions* per unit mass. The old unit of exposure is the *roentgen*. The *SI unit* is the C kg^{-1}.

fission — A process in which a *nucleus* is split into two or more fragments of comparable size.

gamma-radiation (γ-radiation) — Electromagnetic radiation emitted by the *nucleus* as it reverts to its ground state from an excited energy state.

gray (Gy) — The *SI unit* of *absorbed (radiation) dose*. One gray equals 1 J kg^{-1}.

half-life (of a radionuclide) ($T_{\frac{1}{2}}$) — The physical half-life $(T_{\frac{1}{2}})_P$, is the time required for the *activity* of the *radionuclide* to be reduced to one-half of its original value. $(T_{\frac{1}{2}})_P = 0.693/\lambda$. The biological half-life, $(T_{\frac{1}{2}})_B$, is the time required for the activity in the body to be reduced to one-half. If the biological clearance is also exponential, then the effective half-life, $(T_{\frac{1}{2}})_E$, is given by $1/(T_{\frac{1}{2}})_E = 1/(T_{\frac{1}{2}})_P + 1/(T_{\frac{1}{2}})_B$.

half-value layer (of an absorbing material) (HVL) — The thickness required to reduce the intensity of a parallel beam of X- or γ-radiation to one-half. $HVL = 0.693/\mu$ where μ is the linear attenuation coefficient.

internal conversion — A process whereby the energy of a gamma-ray *photon* may be imparted to an inner orbital *electron*, which is then ejected from the *atom*.

ion — A charged *atom* or molecule, that is one which has lost or gained one or more *electrons*. Ions can exist in gases or in solution.

ionising radiations — Radiations which produce ions in the material through which they pass. They may be electromagnetic, as X- or γ-radiation, or particulate, as α- and β-radiation.

isomeric transition — A process whereby an atomic *nucleus* changes from a higher to a lower state of energy, by emitting γ-radiation, with a detectable *half-life*.

isotopes — Nuclides having the same atomic number, but different mass numbers, e.g. ${}^{16}_{8}O$, ${}^{17}_{8}O$ and ${}^{18}_{8}O$ are three isotopes of oxygen.

mass number of a nuclide (A) — The total number of particles, that is *protons* plus *neutrons*, in the *nucleus* of the *atom*.

maximum permissible dose (MPD) — See DEL.

metastable state — Term used to denote a *nuclide* in which the *nucleus* is in an excited state, and decays to its ground state by *isomeric transition*.

neutron — A fundamental uncharged particle of mass 1.675×10^{-27} kg (1.009 m_u). A common constituent of all *nuclei*.

nuclear reactor — A structure in which *neutrons* give rise to a *fission* chain reaction which can be controlled and maintained. *Neutrons* in the reactor may be utilised to irradiate targets for *radionuclide* production.

nucleus — The central part of an *atom* consisting of *protons* and *neutrons*.

nuclide — A species of *atom* with a specific *atomic number* and *mass number*, e.g. ${}^{17}_{8}O$, ${}^{24}_{11}Na$, ${}^{131}_{53}I$.

photon — The unit of electromagnetic radiation, e.g. of light, ultraviolet, X-, or gamma-radiation. Its energy is equal to $h\nu$, where h is Planck's constant (6.626×10^{-34} J s), and ν is the frequency of the radiation (s^{-1}).

positron — A positively charged *electron*, given off during the *radioactive decay* of some nuclei. It is unstable, and in combination with an *electron* it undergoes annihilation to form *annihilation radiation*.

proton — A fundamental particle of mass 1.673×10^{-27} kg (1.007 m_u) and having one unit of positive charge (1.602×10^{-19} C). A common constituent of all *nuclei*.

rad	The old unit of *absorbed (radiation) dose.* One rad equals 10^{-2} J kg^{-1}, i.e. 10^{-2} *gray.*
radioactive decay	The exponential reduction of the number of *atoms* in a radioactive source as it undergoes *disintegration.*
radioactivity	A property of some *nuclides* whereby the *nuclei* disintegrate spontaneously, with the emission or absorption of charged particles or emission of *gamma-radiation.* In charged particle decay the *atoms* are transformed into the atoms of a different element.
radionuclide	A *radioactive nuclide.*
radiopharmaceutical	Any *radioactive* product which is administered to a human being, for medicinal purposes, usually investigational, in which the *radioactivity* is an essential part of the product.
rem	The old unit of *dose equivalent*, with the same dimensions as the *rad.*
roentgen (*R*)	The old unit of *exposure.* One R equals 2.58×10^{-4} C kg^{-1}.
SI units	The International System of Units. The SI units of *activity* and *absorbed dose*, the *becquerel* and the *gray*, were adopted in 1975. The old units, the *curie* and the *rad*, are still in use, but are to be gradually abandoned, together with the *roentgen* and the *rem*, over a period of 5 to 10 years. The following prefixes are used to construct decimal multiples of units:

Multiple	Prefix	Symbol	Multiple	Prefix	Symbol
10^{-1}	deci	d	10	deca	da
10^{-2}	centi	c	10^{2}	hecto	h
10^{-3}	milli	m	10^{3}	kilo	k
10^{-6}	micro	μ	10^{6}	mega	M
10^{-9}	nano	n	10^{9}	giga	G
10^{-12}	pico	p	10^{12}	tera	T
10^{-15}	femto	f	10^{15}	peta	P
10^{-18}	alto	a	10^{18}	exa	E

sievert	The *SI unit* of *dose equivalent.* It has the same dimensions as the *gray.*

Index

G indicates an entry in the Glossary.